Verbotonal Speech Treatment

Verbotonal Speech Treatment

Carl W. Asp, Ph.D.

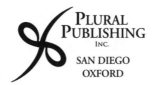

PLURAL
PUBLISHING
INC.

SAN DIEGO
OXFORD

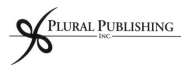

5521 Ruffin Road
San Diego, CA 92123

e-mail: info@pluralpublishing.com
Web site: http://www.pluralpublishing.com

49 Bath Street
Abington, Oxfordshire OX14 1EA
United Kingdom

Typeset in 10/12 Palatino by Flanagan's Publishing Services
Printed in the United States of America by McNaughton and Gunn

ISBN-13: 978-1-59756-046-7
ISBN-10: 1-59756-046-4
Library of Congress Control Number: 2005908641

Contents

Preface

This auditory-based clinical handbook is written as an introduction to the Verbotonal approach. Professor Petar Guberina started the Verbotonal system in 1954 in Zagreb, Croatia. The system included habilitation, rehabilitation, diagnosis, foreign languages, and speech therapy. He used the method as a strategy when working with the hearing impaired. Over the past 51 years (1954–present), the Verbotonal system has been used in over 50 countries in the world.

I have worked closely with Professor Guberina in research and Verbotonal Clinical Workshops in many countries. This close working relationship has allowed me to obtain a thorough understanding of the Verbotonal system.

This handbook has strategies for Vestibular, Auditory, Speech, Second Language, and Treatment Tools/Programs. It is designed for teachers and clinicians in the areas of audiology, speech pathology, special education, education of the deaf, and other related areas. It is intended for use in a Verbotonal course, an aural rehabilitation course, second language learning, and especially for individual use by clinicians and teachers. If all the strategies and treatment tools are used, the clinical results should be excellent. Most children develop have excellent listening skills, intelligible speech, and good voice quality.

Part of the book explains the Verbotonal Auditory Training Units, which is an advanced auditory technology. This technology was first known as SUVAG (System Universal Audition Guberina) units. These units are commercially available through the SUVAG company in France, the Verboton Company in Croatia, and the Listen Company in the United States. All units have similar electroacoustic characteristics and are used with all types of communication disorders and differences.

The handbook explains the Verbotonal approach with a variety of clinical examples. The strategy and the treatment tools are effective. For example, the use of body movements is an indirect way of developing rhythm, intonation, and voice quality patterns and is the basis for effective listening skills and intelligible speech patterns. A glossary of terms is included.

Verbotonal certification is available through the International and National Verbotonal Societies. The international scope of this approach is well developed.

I have changed some of the original Verbotonal terminology, which was developed in the Croat language. For example, the Verbotonal approach is used rather than a system or a method. I hope the newer terminology in English will be acceptable to the reader.

The auditory-based Verbotonal approach is appropriate for the current emphasis in cochlear implants and other auditory technology. It is an exciting time as auditory-based strategies have unlimited potential for helping people with communication disorders and differences.

The reader is free to choose some or all of the treatment tools. My view is that the whole package provides the most effective treatment, but the teacher or clinician should choose what is best for his or her clients.

Professor Carl W. Asp

Acknowledgments

I extend a special thanks to Professor Petar Guberina, who started the Verbotonal System in 1954. His creativity and leadership inspired me and others to contribute to the system.

I thank Professor Claude Roberge and Professor Youngsun Kim, along with Dr. Michelle Cutler for their editorial comments and their encouragement. Also a special thanks to Julie Alspaugh, my graduate assistant, for typing and editing the handbook. Her daily effort was outstanding.

I am grateful for specific contributions to the handbook by Leslee Rook, Julie Alspaugh, G. Aras, Cathy Davis, Allison Dowell, and Professor Youngsun Kim. I also acknowledge Madeline Kline and John Berry for the information they provided.

I thank Ron Holder and Pat Adkinson for their technical assistance in preparing the manuscript. I am grateful to the University students, who field tested the manuscript in my classes, and to all the students who completed the Verbotonal classes.

I thank Knox County, Knoxville, Miami-Dade School System, and the Blount Hearing and Speech Center for implementing the Verbotonal approach. Thanks to the Verbotonal teachers and clinicians throughout the world.

I extend a special thanks to my lovely wife, Jan, who inspired me to develop the handbook. I also thank our five children, Bill, Shannon, Patrick, Kathy, and Jessie, and my sister, Nancy Parker, for their encouragement. This strong family support was a source of inspiration.

CHAPTER

1

Introduction to the Verbotonal Approach

The Verbotonal Approach is an auditory-based strategy that maximizes the listening skills of children and adults who are deaf or hard of hearing, while simultaneously developing intelligible spoken language through binaural listening. The Verbotonal Approach emphasizes a child's auditory perception and speech production of speech rhythm and intonation, which provides the foundation for developing good listening skills and intelligible speech.

Knox County Schools in Tennessee and Miami-Dade Public Schools in Florida have both successfully adapted the Verbotonal Approach to their school curriculum. Listening skills and spoken language skills are taught throughout the entire school day. These skills help the children have access to regular classrooms in the least restricted environment. Clinicians who are competent in error analysis and utilization of the treatment tools can implement an effective treatment plan for each child. Parents are included in all phases of their child's development.

This book reviews the Verbotonal Approach history, strategy, treatment tools, sequencing, and programs in action. The Vestibular, Auditory, Speech, and Second Language treatment strategies of the Verbotonal Approach are presented as the author's interpretation of the Verbotonal Approach to intervention; this might vary slightly from the view of other Verbotonalists.

1

The Verbotonal Approach began in 1939 in Croatia, when Professor Petar Guberina developed an auditory-based strategy for teaching foreign languages through well-developed listening skills. In 1954, Guberina expanded this auditory strategy to serve children and adults with hearing impairments and other communication problems. He identified it as the Verbotonal Approach. In 1963, the author joined Professor Guberina to develop clinical research programs using the Verbotonal Approach in the United States (Asp & Guberina, 1981). The main goal of the Verbotonal Approach is to maximize the listening skills of children and adults who are deaf or hard of hearing, while simultaneously developing good spoken language through binaural speech stimulation.

With this goal in mind, a Verbotonal Auditory Training Unit was constructed to advance the listening skills of each child and adult. Consisting of a binaural headset, filters, and a wrist vibrator, this unit enables the child to simultaneously feel and hear the clinician's speech model, their classmates' response, and their own speech. This training unit facilitates the child's adjustment to his personal hearing aids or cochlear implant by highlighting his residual hearing and correcting his speech errors through listening.

For children with profound hearing losses, researchers have consistently demonstrated that children with cochlear implants have higher performance in speech perception and production than children with hearing aids (Osberger, Robbin, Todd, Riley, & Miyamoto, 1994; Tobey, Geers, & Brenner, 1994). However, Pisoni et al. (2000) reported that some implant users are "stars" while others do not reach their potential. This suggested that the listening skills of the less successful implant users were not fully developed, and a more effective listening strategy was needed. Establishing an effective listening strategy is also important for individuals with multiple handicaps, such as having a vestibular weakness in addition to cochlear damage (Guberina, 1972). The vestibular weakness can be addressed by targeting body movements as part of the child's spoken language development.

Young, normal-hearing children process meaningful speech through feeling, hearing, and seeing; a multisensory input that results in sensory integration (Ayres, 1978). Through sensory integration, the neuroplasticity of the child's brain develops new neural pathways and expands his learning potential (Ryugo et al., 2000). The Verbotonal Approach is based on the neuroplasticity of the child's brain, especially during the critical language-learning period. It is designed to provide the important link between the child's auditory cortex (auditory) and associated sensory areas (vestibular and speech); or in simple terms, the link between the child's brain, body, and tongue. The strategy is to gradually change from a multisensory (feeling, hearing, touching, and seeing) to a unisensory (auditory) speech input by reducing the visual and tactile cues without frustrating the child or adult. This change to unisensory auditory input occurs more quickly with higher-level auditory skills, possibly with a cochlear implant.

This book is based on the authors' clinical experience, insights, and ongoing research in the Verbotonal Approach. The purpose of this book is to present a therapeutic strategy to improve the auditory and speech skills of children and adults with hearing losses (Asp & Guberina, 1981; Asp, 1985). The Verbotonal Approach is currently used in some public schools, private clinics, and University programs in the United States as well as in many other countries (e.g., France, Spain, Italy, Russia, Brazil, Senegal, Egypt, Japan, Taiwan, etc.).

The Verbotonal Approach is divided into Vestibular, Auditory, Speech, and Second Language strategies and their corresponding treatment tools. These tools highlight the child's rhythm and speech patterns, for they are the foundation of both listening and speaking skills. Although the discussion follows the order listed, the application of the tools is done simultaneously in treatment. For example, the child wears a binaural hearing headset (part of the Verbotonal Auditory Training Unit) while the clinician stimulates him with body movements (vestibular) and speech modifications (speech). Because sequencing is important, a separate section describes how the tools are used in sequence.

The book is written using the "clinician" as the provider of treatment; "clinician" may refer to teachers, therapists, and so forth. The child or adult receiving treatment is often referred to as "he" throughout the book, and "mother" is assigned as the child's caretaker. These generalizations are not made to offend or overlook anyone; they are used to simplify the explanations and maintain consistency throughout the book.

The History of Body Movements and Vestibular Exercises

In 1954, Professor Guberina applied his auditory-based strategy for teaching foreign language (French, Spanish, Italian, etc.) to improve the auditory perception of adults with hearing impairments. He used acoustic filters to highlight the vowels and consonants needed for correct perception. He named this approach the Verbotonal Approach (System).

In 1957, Professor Guberina expanded this auditory strategy to children who were deaf or hard of hearing. These children needed daily stimulation of rhythm and intonation patterns, which was implemented in groups of eight to ten children. Body movements were added to his treatment strategy by combining his phonetic theory with Rudolph Laban's theory of the movements for dance. Laban was a famous Hungarian dancer who applied the efficient and elegant movements of workers performing daily tasks to his dance program. In conjunction with Laban's Dance Program, Guberina developed a body movement program.

To implement his strategy, Professor Guberina worked with Ms. Vesna Pintar, a Croatian ballet dancer, who was studying the relationship between phonetics and movement at Zagreb University. Together they constructed a videotape demonstration in which each vowel had an optimal body movement for stimulation. For example, while phonating the vowel /i/, Ms. Pintar moved both of her arms above her waist to create more tension; whereas for the vowel /a/, she opened both arms at waist level, creating less tension. In 1975, in the United States, the writer of this book and his clinical associate modified these body movements to be either parameter-based or phoneme-based (Asp, 1985). As an example, for the parameter-based stimulation of duration, the clinician moves her arms horizontally in harmony with a long /a/ followed by a short /a/. For phoneme-stimulation of /a/, she would open both arms while phonating the vowel /a/. The parameter stimulus and phoneme stimulus are similar, because the movements are less tense and move on a horizontal plane; only the emphasis differs. The clinician chooses either to concentrate on a specific parameter or on a specific phoneme.

References

Asp, C. W. (1985). The Verbotonal method for management of young hearing impaired children. *Ear and Hearing, 6*(1), 39–42.

Asp, C. W., & Guberina, P. (1981). *Verbotonal method for rehabilitating people with communication problems*. New York: NY: World Rehabilitation Fund, Inc.

Ayres, A. J. (1978). Learning disabilities and the vestibular system. *Journal of Learning Disabilities, 11*, 18–29.

Guberina, P. (1972). *The correlation between sensitivity of the vestibular system, and hearing and speech in verbotonal rehabilitation* (Appendix 6, pp. 256–260). Washington, DC: Office of Vocational Rehabilitation, Department of Health, Education, and Welfare.

Osberger, M. J., Robbins, A. M., Todd, S. L., Riley, A. I., & Miyamoto, R. T. (1994). Speech production skills of children with multichannel cochlear implants. In I. J. Hochmair-Desoyer & E. S. Hochmair (Eds.), *Advances in cochlear implants* (pp. 503–508). Wien, Germany: Manz.

Pisoni, B. D., Cleary, M. C., Geers, A. E., & Tobey, E. A. (2000). Individual differences in effectiveness of cochlear implants in children who are prelingually deaf; new process measures of performance. *Volta Review, 101*(3), 111–164.

Ryugo, D., Limb, C., & Redd, E. (2000). Brain plasticity. In J. K. Niparko, K. I. Kirk, N. K. Mellon, A. M. Robbins, D. L. Tucci, & B.S. Wilson (Eds.), *Cochlear implants* (pp. 33–56). Philadelphia, PA: Lippincott Williams & Wilkins.

Tobey, E., Geers, A. E., & Brenner, C. (1994). Speech production results; speech feature acquisition. *Volta Review, 96,* 109–129.

CHAPTER

2

Vestibular Strategy: Vocalize While Moving

During the preword stage a normally developing infant-toddler moves his body freely while he vocalizes. The child's vestibular system coordinates and creates a harmony for motor speech feedback simultaneously through tactile, proprioceptive, auditory, and speech input (Figure 2–1). The motor coordination and control begins with whole body movements, and then later includes oral-motor speech control.

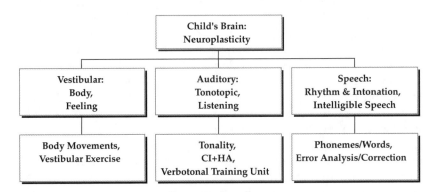

Figure 2–1. The Brain's Link Between the Vestibular, Auditory, and Speech Input

In short, while the child is listening, he learns effective oral-motor speech control with the help of his body.

The changes in muscle tone and tension over time are part of a normal child's development of motor skills. He first crawls, then walks, then runs, and so forth. These movements are accompanied by vocalizations. The larger body movements create a strong link among the child's body, tongue, and ears. For example, an increase in overall body tension directly affects the fine muscle tension of the tongue, vocal folds, and other speech articulators, because both the body and the articulators are in harmony. As the normal oral-motor speech patterns are established, they provide a foundation for later speech pattern processing and control.

Standard vestibular exercises provide a multisensory input, including touch, proprioception, hearing, and vision (Aras, 2000; Palmer, 1999; Pansini, 2000; Fisher et al., 1991). These exercises help develop gross motor (body) skills such as crawling, creeping, toe-to-heel walking, and so forth; and they are based on the motor milestones of normally developing children (Palmer, 1999). For children with hearing impairments, some researchers have reported deficits in motor skills, such as balance and fast, complex movements (Ayres, 1978; Guberina, 1972; Horak et al, 1988). The vestibular exercises in the Verbotonal Approach has the child vocalize in harmony with each movement in the exercise. For example, the clinician produces the syllable /pa/ with each step of her toe-to-heel walking. Then the children, one by one, imitate the clinician's model of phonation and toe-to-heel walking. The simultaneous vocal phonation and body movement allows the child to practice speech and motor control in harmony.

Once the children can control their bodies while walking in a straight line, the treatment can progress to whole-body speech movements with the children standing or sitting in a half-circle around the clinician (Asp, 1985; Asp & Guberina, 1981; Sussman, 1996). These body movements are designed to strengthen the body's link to the child's phonation, and to help him develop a natural-sounding voice quality. The clinician uses the seven speech parameters; which include rhythm, intonation, tension, pause, duration, loudness, and pitch, for both stimulation and indirect correction. For example, the clinician moves while vocalizing the syllables /ma ma ma ma (pause) ma/. This many-to-one rhythmic syllable pattern highlights the parameters of rhythm, pause, and tension. Vocalization with whole-body movements helps the child gain control of the length and tempo of his vocal patterns and use speech pauses effectively. As his motor memory develops, he will be able to produce this speech rhythm by himself, without the clinician providing a model.

The vestibular body movements are considered indirect stimulation of speech production, because the child's attention is on the body movements and not on the speech mechanism. This strategy allows for a more natural means of shaping the child's speech production. The seven speech parameters can be highlighted separately using body movements, but most are linked with other speech parameters. For example, the clinician raises her arms with a wide sweeping motion while phonating /i/, forcing her vocalization to go from a low to a high vocal pitch level. As the child imitates the clinician, his overall body tension increases, which helps him perceive and produce a rising intonation pattern. If the child needs more speech input, he wears a wrist vibrator so he can feel the rising intonation pattern. The seven speech parameters, taught through body movements and vibrotactile feedback, are effective for establishing the preword rhythm and intonation speech patterns as a foundation for his listening (auditory) skills.

Once accurate speech pattern perception is established, the body movements become more phoneme-based and emphasize the individual phonemes within the coarticulation patterns of speech. For example, a tense muscular body movement is used while vocalizing the tense vowel /i/ and a less tense body movement is used to emphasize the less tense vowel /a/. The nasal consonant /m/ requires a longer body movement with less tension, whereas the short nasal /n/ needs the opposite. With a falling intonation pattern, the initial prevocalic consonant has more tension than the final postvocalic consonant. These tension differences help to develop accurate perception and production of coarticulated speech patterns.

On the practical side, the modified vestibular exercises and the body movements are effective with infants, toddlers, and preschoolers, because they are fun and meaningful to young children. When used with a small group of preschoolers, the friendly peer competition keeps the children vocalizing and alert throughout the entire session. Movements can be adapted for individual treatment of different ages and motoric levels. For example, a clinician moves an infant's legs while he babbles. A toddler, who can sit upright, receives a similar stimulation with his arms. Finally, when the child can stand independently, the movements involve the whole body, and the child initiates his own movements in imitation. These body movements can be carried over to the home environment once the parents have received special training from the clinician.

Both the body (vestibular system) and the ear (auditory system) provide information for the brain to process and verbalize speech (Figure 2–1). Developmentally, the body is the dominant sensory input for the fetus and infant, through the feeling of movements and skin contacts. Later, the sensory inputs are unified, and the ear (auditory system) becomes the dominant sense for perceiving and producing speech.

Motoric milestones are developmental milestones that most young children achieve at each age level. These milestones allow for comparison with a group standard of motor development. For example, crawling is mastered by young infants at nine months of age, whereas toe-to-heel walking is established at four years of age.

The Link: Body, Tongue, and Ear

The vestibular system's primary function is the perception of the body movements (position, acceleration, deceleration) in space and the effects of gravity on the child's body. In the periphery, the vestibular organ is part of the inner ear, where it is connected with the cochlea, sharing the same phylogenetic and embryologic origin. The sense of hearing extended from the vestibular perception of feeling. Now both function in harmony for the simultaneous feeling and hearing of speech (Aras & Asp, 2005).

In the periphery, both organs (vestibular organ and cochlea) are stimulated by the rhythm and intonation changes through the low-frequency speech patterns. The sacculus, within the vestibular end-organ, is sensitive to low-frequency speech rhythm. For example, while in his mother's uterus, an infant feels the speech rhythm of his mother's vocal patterns. He continues to feel these speech rhythms after he is born when his mother holds him closely. By feeling these speech rhythms, he begins to develop his proprioceptive memory; this provides a foundation for the later development of auditory memory. In short, what he "feels" early on, he later "hears" (Aras & Asp, 2005).

As with the cochlea, the central part of the vestibular system is even more important than the peripheral system. It serves as an integrator and organizer for all the senses for space perception; first in the brainstem, and later in the cortex. This is why we exercise and stimulate vestibular perception: to unify all sensory input through the child's body. The neuroplasticity within the nervous system develops new synapses and links with other neurons when both vestibular exercises and body movements are performed in harmony with vocalization. This allows the speech rhythms to be perceived through both proprioception and the vestibular end-organ (Aras & Asp, 2005).

Vestibular Processing of Speech

As mentioned previously, the link between the body, the tongue, and the ear is established through the brain's plasticity. The muscular generalization allows the muscular tension of the peripheral muscle groups during body movements to be automatically transferred to the inner muscle groups of the tongue, mandible, maxilla, and vocal cords. The child feels the speech rhythm but is unaware of these specific associated developments. In summary, the child's body develops an overall orientation in space through simultaneous body movements and vocal patterns.

The Vestibular System

Vestibulocochlear Hearing

Because of the close proximity of the vestibular end-organ and the cochlea, the Verbotonal Approach develops the vestibular system's role in hearing (Figure 2–1). The child's brain is sensitive to a broad bandwidth, 2 to 20,000 Hz. The vestibular end-organ responds acoustically from 2 to 1000 Hz, while the cochlea responds to speech energy between 20 and 20,000 Hz. These two organs overlap in the 20 to 1,000 Hz frequency range. The vestibular and auditory systems both process the rhythm and intonation patterns of speech below 300 Hz, whereas the cochlea is "tuned" to the tonalities of the 43 phonemes above 300 Hz. The Verbotonal Auditory Training Unit has the capacity to help the child develop these specific perceptions. It will be explained in more detail later in the text.

Vestibular and Balance Assessment

Because the vestibular system is integral to the Verbotonal Approach, an accurate diagnosis of vestibular function is important. Whenever possible, the assessment should include testing with electronystagmography (ENG) and a stabilometer. The ENG measures the fast and slow phase of each eye movement for body rotation or caloric stimulation (warm or cold water), or from a series of lights in a dark room. The movements of the child's eyes from these stimulations are a measurement of how his peripheral and central vestibular system functions.

The stabilometry is used with an older child. The child stands on a platform that is calibrated; the movement of the platform measures the child's balance. If the child has good balance, he will reorient himself quickly when the platform is tilted. If the child does not have good balance, he will not be able to adjust his position quickly enough; he will lose his balance and possibly fall (Aras & Asp, 2005).

Other assessment procedures include a motor test that is administered by a physical therapist, occupational therapist, or otolaryngologist. The motor test involves walking toe-to-heel on balance beams of different lengths and widths, as well as motor movements such as crawling, creeping, and skipping. These tests are part of a standard assessment, the Vestibular Exercises Test Battery, or a specific test such as the Ozeresky test, or a test within the Peabody Language Test. The results of the motor test are compared to the motor milestones of infants, toddlers, and young children with normal hearing. Each test has age-appropriate norms for the developmental level of the child. A comparison to the norms provides useful information about the child's motoric level relative to his peers (Aras & Asp, 2005).

Vestibular Weakness: Balance and Coordination Problems

When a 50 dB or greater hearing loss is present, the child's vestibular sensitivity and balance usually indicate weakness or a reduced level of sensitivity. Therefore, a child with a profound hearing loss (+90 dB HL) has a greater incidence of vestibular damage. In the United States, most audiologists and physicians do not typically evaluate the child's vestibular sensitivity, space perception, or motoric skills. However, the Verbotonal Hearing and Speech Center in Zagreb, Croatia completes a vestibular assessment on all children with disabilities.

Reduced sensitivity can also occur in children with normal hearing. Children with severe language disorders, central auditory processing disorder (CAPD), attention deficit disorder (ADD), attention deficit hyperactivity disorder (ADHD), learning disability (LD), and so forth often have difficulty processing the rhythm and intonation patterns of speech, have a reduced auditory memory, and may demonstrate vestibular weakness.

Even though a child may have a weak vestibular system with or without a hearing loss, the neuroplasticity of the child's brain will develop new dendrite connections. The brain (central nervous system) compensates for the peripheral vestibular weakness. This compensation is facilitated by the Vestibular Strategy of the Verbotonal Approach, which emphasizes vestibular exercises and body movements with phonation to improve the child's motoricity, orientation in space, and memory span. Both the body (vestibular system) and the ear (auditory system) provide sensory information to the child's brain for processing and verbalizing speech, so both are an important part of the Verbotonal Approach.

The Body and Space Perception

As previously mentioned, the fetus develops a three-dimensional (3D) perception of space, spacioception, by moving in the mother's womb. The early experience serves as the foundation for his 3D space perception after birth. As the infant develops, his space perception expands. The development of space perception involves input from the five organs: (1) touch, (2) proprioception, (3) vestibular sense, (4) hearing, and (5) sight; it is a multisensory input.

The highest level of processing and verbalizing speech is space grammar. At the preword (prelinguistic) level, space grammar is the temporal arrangement of the child's babbling of a series of syllables as a speech pattern. This arrangement of syllables provides the foundation for the grammatic rules for the syntax of a natural spoken language. These speech syllables occur in space over time. The infant uses cooing, babbling, vocalized emotions, and imitations to create a speech jargon that is not intelligible to most adults, but this jargon follows the appropriate speech rhythms of the suprasegmentals. If the child has a weak link between his speech production and his perception, he is usually delayed in producing these basic speech patterns. As the infant internalizes the grammar rules, he will begin to produce more word combinations and his space grammar expands to the word and sentence level.

Tactile and Proprioceptive Memory

The sensory input of touch (feeling) is an important modality for both the perception and production of speech. The feeling from body movements and touch includes the speech articulators, for example, the tongue, teeth, velum, and so forth. As the tongue moves through the oral cavity to form different coarticulation patterns, the child receives tactile and proprioceptive input to develop his memory patterns.

The proprioceptive input to the brain comes from the awareness of the body's weight, posture, movement, and position in space. This is closely related to the awareness and perception of the state (position) of the child's limbs and body postures. For example, with eyes closed, a child visualizes the location and movement of his index finger with his arm extended. In parallel, a similar perception occurs in the child's oral cavity. For example, proprioception of the postures and movement of the tongue and lips for the coarticulation of a series of phonemes; this helps the child develop proprioceptive memory. If the child has a hearing impairment, the link to auditory perception is weak and he is unable to develop intelligible speech without specialized treatment.

Proprioceptive memory of five to ten syllables provides the "memory map" in the child's brain. With this "memory map," the child can verbalize normal speech patterns that have up to fifteen phonemes per second. These proprioceptive maps are also used as the foundation for developing the child's auditory memory. As an analogy, "Name That Tune" was a television game show for remembering well-known songs. Some contestants named the correct song by hearing only the first two musical notes of the songs. This highly refined memory skill was developed during childhood by singing along with others on a regular basis with a high emotional level. This repetitious singing provided the foundation for the child's auditory memory. Then, later as a young adult, he is able to recall his favorite songs by hearing only the first two notes of the song. This proprioceptive feedback provides the foundation for refined auditory memory.

Muscular Generalization

The Verbotonal Approach is based on how infants and toddlers move while vocalizing. Their movements and vocalizations are linked and are in harmony with one another. For example, if the infant has a long vocalization, he simultaneously uses a long body movement. If his vocal pattern is short and quick, his body movement is short and quick. The child's body movements affect the quality of his oral motor speech patterns; this is referred to as muscular generalization.

Muscular generalization is used to describe how the child's body movements affect motor speech patterns and is the underlying principle of using body movements as a treatment tool. For example, after eating, the infant's body is very relaxed, so he moves his limbs slowly. He lowers his vocal pitch with the less tense vowel /a/ and the less tense consonant /m/. His babbling would be /ma ma ma ma/, with the least tension possible, for he is relaxed and content. In contrast, if he is very hungry or tired, both his body tension and vocal pitch increase and his movements are short, quick, and very tense, such as /Λ Λ Λ Λ/ while crying.

As another example of muscular generalization, a child who has "clonic block" during stuttering will repeat the vowel /o/ of the first syllable in "Oh Boy," and have difficulty shifting to the word "boy." His repetitive vocal production of /o/ will create excessive tension in both his body and vocal cords. If he decreases his body tension, his vocal tension will also decrease, and he will be able to coarticulate the words, "Oh Boy." The decrease in vocal tension is necessary for a smooth coarticulated speech pattern moving from one syllable or phoneme to the next. This is called "loose contact" in stuttering therapy.

As mentioned previously, muscular generalization is the basic principle of using body movements as a treatment tool to improve speech perception and production. The movements indirectly affect the child's articulation and vocalization patterns and enhance proprioceptive memory. For example, a long horizontal arm movement from far right to far left is used in coordination with the vocalization of the sustained vowel, /a/. This is considered indirect stimulation because the child is unaware of how his vocal patterns are changing; he is mainly focused on imitating the clinician's body movements.

Indirect stimulation of the child's vocal patterns with body movements is an effective strategy for developing the natural rhythm and intonation of speech and natural voice quality. This indirect movement strategy is in contrast to the Phonetic Placement Strategy, which uses a mirror to show the child how to place his tongue and lips to produce an individual speech sound. Phonetic placement is a strategy that assumes the child can remember one articulation position after another position in a series of speech sounds, such as fifteen phonemes in one second. In contrast, the Verbotonal Approach uses indirect stimulation of body movements to teach the coarticulation of phonemes in a sequential pattern.

Because young children enjoy body movements, an effective clinician can conduct a two-hour body movement session with a group of eight three-year-old children. This treatment strategy, which incorporates simultaneous movement and vocalization, is fun and natural for an infant, toddler, or a young child. Even a fetus moves arms, legs, and head in his mother's womb to the feeling and sounds of his mother's voice. A young infant continues to move and vocalize at the same time as part of normal motor development. Movement also stimulates overall growth and coordination.

In contrast to children who are constantly in motion, most adults sit more than they stand or move around. For example, an adult clinician uses an adult therapy model for young children when she and the child are seated in chairs, with no body movements. This typical adult-based therapy plan is not fun or appropriate for young children, because it is difficult for them to sit for extended periods of time and to carryover what was practiced during the session to other environments.

With the Verbotonal Approach, the clinician does not use chairs when providing therapy to young children; rather she starts on the floor and introduces body movements to indirectly control the child's vocal pattern and tongue movements. This is more fun for both the clinician and the young child; it motivates both of them and helps to develop the child's self-confidence in imitating the clinician's speech patterns.

The body movements that are performed in conjunction with the vocal and articulation patterns provide simultaneous input into the child's brain. This helps to develop his proprioceptive memory so that he can achieve the appropriate motor milestones. The child automatically uses his "motor maps" to remember how to verbalize the appropriate rhythm, intonation, and phonemic patterns of speech.

In speech production, the child's brain simultaneously processes body movements and the movement of the articulators from both tactile and proprioceptive feedback. To perceive the speech patterns of others, the body functions as a resonator. For example, the child "feels" lower pitched sounds in his abdomen, which resonates lower frequencies, such as the vowel /a/ (below 800 Hz). Higher pitched sounds such as the consonant /s/ (at 6000 Hz) are "felt" in the head, which is tuned to higher pitched sounds. Functioning as a resonator, the child's body provides feedback to help the child perceive the speech patterns of others.

The vibrotactile speech input from the speech vibrator on the Verbotonal Auditory Training Unit assists the child feel the clinician's vocal rhythm through his body while hearing her speech sounds through the headsets. Vibrotactile speech input helps the child perceive and produce speech in harmony with his body movements and those of the clinician.

Vestibular Habilitation

The goal of auditory habilitation is to maximize the feeling and hearing of speech rhythm. As mentioned earlier, these "feelings" are targeted through body movements, along with simultaneous vibratory input from a speech vibrator. The speech vibrator on the Verbotonal Auditory Training Unit is first used with a "sounding board," on which the infant lays or sits. The young child feels the vocalized speech rhythm through his whole body, while he vocalizes.

Later, a speech vibrator that is more localized is placed on the infant/toddler; it is usually placed on the child's wrist or ankle. The speech vibrator provides vibrotactile input that coordinates with the speech dialogue between the child and his or her mother or clinician.

This helps to facilitate the child's, perception and production of speech rhythms. The speech vibrator accomplishes the same feedback as a mother who holds her child closely while she vocalizes. The child can feel and perceive the speech rhythms as they are produced.

Treatment with a young infant or toddler includes simultaneous vestibular (movement), auditory (listening), and speech (production) stimulation. For example, body tension increases by raising the arms while voicing or by pushing one hand against the other while voicing (isometric tension). Both examples increase body tension, but they look different to the child visually. The clinician emphasizes an increase in body tension and not a particular movement. When the child stabilizes his production and perception, he articulates the correct phoneme without needing the assistance of a body movement.

Vestibular Exercises in Space: Vocalize While Moving

With the Verbotonal Approach, movements are used progressively, beginning with vestibular exercises while moving in a straight line and progressing to controlled body movements within an established circle. The vestibular exercises are based on the infant/toddler's maturity and balance skills. These include walking forward and backward (toe-to-heel on a beam or line on the floor), side-to-side, rolling over onto the back, running, skipping, and so forth. The vestibular exercises are typically used by physical or occupational therapists to develop the child's motor skills and balance. The level of the child's motor skills (motor patterns) is related to the child's rhythm and speech patterns. As the child's motor skills improve, perception and production of speech patterns improve as well. When the Verbotonal clinician uses vestibular exercise, she vocalizes with each movement to enhance the child's memory patterns.

Verbotonal Vestibular Exercises

In the Verbotonal Speech and Hearing Center in Zagreb, the Verbotonal clinician uses the vestibular exercises to develop the child's balance, to establish an input to the central monitoring system, and to increase the vestibular input for space perception. These exercises are physical games that are within the child's physical potential. These exercises include jumping rope, changing positions or directions while swinging, walking on a balance beam with eyes open or closed, turning around in each direction, turning on a cross bar, rolling forward and backward on the floor, and jumping to complete a circle in two to four jumps. These vestibular exercises are presented in three levels of complexity.

Level 1 is an analytic strategy, using each of the five senses. New exercises are gradually introduced until the child has difficulty with them. Later, when the child's performance has improved, the same difficult exercises are reintroduced. Although exercises are used for vision, hearing, proprioception, and touch, the exercises for the vestibular sense are the most important.

In Level 2 all the senses are stimulated simultaneously. In the beginning only a few senses are stimulated, but as the child progresses, stimulation of the other senses are added. This is a gradual buildup of stimulation.

Level 3 is the global strategy where the exercises are used to develop the child's automatic motor behavior that he uses in his daily life. Because the strategy is to unify his sensory input, the vestibular exercises enhance his ability to restructure his automatic motor behavior and generalize these skills to everyday life. All the vestibular exercises involve simultaneous phonation during the movement. The combination of moving and phonating helps establish the proprioceptive memory patterns of movement.

The SMART Curriculum

Physical and occupational therapists use many different vestibular programs or curriculums to develop the motor milestones in young children, depending on the level of each child. For example, early-stage milestones include creeping and crawling, whereas later milestones include more controlled movements, such as walking toe-to-heel on a beam. The beam-walking requires a high level of balance, coordination, and strength. These gross motor milestones are followed by fine motor movements, such as holding a pencil and writing the letters of the alphabet.

The Stimulating Maturity through Accelerated Readiness Training (SMART) (Palmer, 1999) curriculum is one such specific vestibular program. It is currently used in the Knox County School System by physical and occupational therapists to develop motor milestones. This curriculum is required for all kindergarten and first grade students. By developing control of their bodies in space and reaching motor milestones, the children are prepared to sit and attend to table activities and instruction for longer periods of time.

The SMART (Palmer, 1999) curriculum is also used by clinicians who are implementing the Verbotonal Approach for children with hearing impairments. The clinician has each child vocalize while moving to develop his proprioceptive memory of rhythm and intonation speech patterns.

In-Line Movements

In the beginning, vestibular movements in a straight line are targeted. Later, movements are performed in a circle. The clinician's first level is on-off stimulation, where the young children run when the clinician vocalizes and "freeze" when the clinician stops. Each child feels the clinician's vocalization through the speech vibrator; the child runs because he feels the speech patterns. Once the child is successful at the on-off level, he progresses to a many-to-one syllable rhythm, as explained earlier /ma ma ma ma (pause) ma/. The children run with slow steps for /ma ma ma/, then pause and produce one controlled movement for the last /ma/. This is the first rhythm the child learns, he goes from many uncontrolled syllables to one controlled syllable. A base drum can also be used to teach this basic rhythm. The low frequency of the drum is easily felt by all the children; they learn to move to the rhythm of the drumbeat. The drumbeat serves as a similar stimulation as the whole body movements for establishing this basic rhythm pattern.

Circle Movements

Body movements within a circle of children who are facing the clinician require a higher level of body stimulation, because each child stands or sits in one place. This requires more body control in space. Some clinician have each child stand or sit on their own carpet square to keep them organized and in order. At this level both parameter-based and phoneme-based stimulation are used and all movements progress from the preword level to the word level to the sentence level.

Typically, with a circle of young children, the clinician begins by using sitting body movements. The clinician uses only the upper part of her body for most of the movements; however, leg movements can be added, such as pulling one leg from a straight to bent position. In each position change she vocalizes in short bursts with the same timing as her movements. The children imitate each movement and vocalization the clinician makes. As the children gain more coordination, motor skill, and confidence, the clinician uses standing body movements. The results of the standing movements are similar to those of the sitting movements.

Body Movements in Space: Vocalize While Moving

Parameter-Based Body Movements

The clinician begins using body movements that are based on parameter stimulation to establish rhythm and intonation patterns. The parameter of duration (e.g., long vs. short movements) is usually a good starting point. She moves her right arm horizontally from far-right to far-left while producing the sustained vowel, /a/. Next, she changes her duration from a long movement with a long vocalization of /a/ to a short duration of movement and vocalization of /ʌ/. Next, she phonates a series of short vowels, /ʌʌʌʌ/, with quick arm movements to highlight changes in syllable rate and the shorter syllable duration (200 msec rather than 400 msec).

The clinician targets the development of intonation patterns with her body movements by changing her muscle tension over time. The children imitate her movements and phonation patterns. For example, she begins with a waist-level movement for /a/ and moves to an above-the-waist movement as her muscle tension and intonation increase in a low-to-high vocal pitch (e.g., 200 Hz to 400 Hz). The intonation change can be long and gradual or short and quick depending on her body movement. In contrast, a downward body movement with a decrease in muscle tension is used for a falling intonation pattern. To elicit this pattern, the clinician begins with a movement above her waist with a high level of tension and then moves below waist level as her tension decreases and her intonation pattern falls (e.g., 400 Hz to 200 Hz).

Table 2–1 displays the perceptual parameters in the middle column. An increase of tension is in the left column and a decrease in tension in the right column. For the parameter of duration, the movement and tension would be short for more tension and long for less tension. The syllable rate would be fast (8 syllables per second) for more tension and slow (3 syllables per second) for less tension. For rhythm, the stressed syllable has more tension relative to the unstressed syllable. Also, more tension is needed to sustain a long pause, whereas a short pause requires less tension because of the quick release of the pause.

The Seven Perceptual Parameters

The organization of the three-dimensional body movements in space includes the horizontal (left-right), vertical (up-down), and depth (back-front) axes. These three axes are used to define different body positions while standing, sitting, or lying on the floor. At the beginning,

Table 2–1. Perceptual Parameters/Phonetic Placement as a Function of Tension for Body Movements

To Increase Tension	Perceptual Parameters	To Decrease Tension
Rising	Intonation	Falling
Stressed syllable	Rhythm	Unstressed syllable
Loud	Loudness	Soft
Short	Duration	Long
Fast	Rate	Slow
Long	Pause with Tension	Short
High	Tonality: (Frequency Zones)	Low
	Phonetic Placement	
Voiceless	Voiced/Voiceless	Voiced
Closed	Vowel Features: (Open/Close)	Open
Initial Syllable Position	Syllable Placement	Final Syllable Position

lying on the floor and sitting positions are used with infants and toddlers. Later, when the children's motor skills and balance are more developed, a standing position is more appropriate. The following is a short explanation of the seven perceptual parameters.

1. **Tension**—The clinician increases her muscle tension by moving her limbs (arms and/or legs) away from their normal state of rest. The "away position" can be up or down, and/or out or in. The clinician can also increase tension with isometric pressure of one hand against the other or against a stationary object, such as a wall. This increase in tension is achieved by an increase in resistance to movement. To create less tension, the clinician moves from the point of greatest tension to the point of least tension through space, moving closer to her state of rest. Tension is the dominant parameter of body movements because it constitutes a physical change in position over time. Collectively, an increase in body movement tension results in an increase in vocal loudness, shorter duration, faster vocal rate, longer vocal pauses, higher tonality, and an overall stressed vocal syllable. In contrast, a decrease in body movement tension collectively results in a softer vocalization, longer vocal duration, slower vocal rate, a shorter pause, a lower tonality, and an overall unstressed vocal syllable. Table 2–1 shows the tension

changes of body movements and vocal patterns for the different perceptual parameters.

2. **Intonation**—The intonation parameter closely follows the tension parameter. Raising her right arm with a wide sweeping motion while phonating /a/ forces the clinician's vocal pitch to reach a high pitch; this represents an upward intonation pattern. For falling vocal pitch (falling intonation pattern), her body movements go from more to less tense with her right arm moving downward. To create a sustained vocal pitch, she moves her arm right-to-left with no change in tension. In the beginning, most children who are deaf start with a monotone pitch. This is not pleasant for the listener, so the clinician needs to change her muscle tension to develop a wide range of intonation patterns to make the child's speech patterns meaningful.

3. **Pitch**—Spectral pitch (tonality) is phoneme-based and is unique to each of the 43 American phonemes (14 vowels, 5 diphthongs, and 24 consonants). Each of these phonemes has a specific spectral pitch in an utterance. For example, the utterance "a mama" has two phonemes, /a/ and /m/. The /m/ is a low-tonality consonant, whereas the /a/ is a mid-tonality vowel.

4. **Duration**—The clinician targets the duration parameter by using left-to-right or right-to left horizontal movement at waist level; for example, moving right-to-left while phonating /a/. The long vs. short duration is represented by moving the arm in harmony with the long vowel /a/ vs. the short vowel /ʌ/. Changing from a fast tempo (/pʌpʌpʌpʌ/) to a slow tempo (/pa—pa—pa—pa/) is distinguished on the same horizontal plane but with different rates of movement and muscular tension.

5. **Pause**—The clinician uses the "pause" parameter by moving in a horizontal plane and initiating/stopping her body movements in harmony with her vocalizations. During the pause there is an increase in tension, and a quick release in tension occurs in the syllable following the pause. A pause can be short (200 msec) or long (500 msec), depending on the speech rhythm pattern. Regardless of the duration of the pause, a pause is always marked with an increase in body and vocal tension.

6. **Loudness**—The clinician demonstrates an increase in vocal loudness (e.g., 65 to 75 dB SPL) with an upward movement of her right arm and a decrease in vocal loudness (e.g., 65 to 55 dB SPL) with a downward, relaxed movement of her right arm. Both of the previ-

ous examples represent a 10 dB variation, but in opposite directions of loudness. The direction of the change is indicated by the direction of the arm movement. As a general rule, the loudness level is greater in stressed syllables than in unstressed syllables.

7. **Rhythm**—The rhythm parameter includes all the above parameters. The clinician's speech rhythm is the global, dominant parameter that the child's brain perceives and remembers as a rhythmic change over time. The clinician's speech rhythm stimulates and helps to develop the child's proprioceptive and auditory memory span.

Phoneme-Based Movements

To understand phoneme-based movement stimulation using the Vestibular Strategy, we should review the well-known vowel diagram that appears in all phonetic textbooks. This vowel diagram is based on an x-ray of the left side of the vocal tract that determined the tongue and jaw positions when each vowel is produced with sustained phonation. This diagram is organized into two dimension: the horizontal dimension of front-central-back orientation, and the vertical dimension of high (closed) to low (open) positions. For speech production, the vowel /i/ is a high-front-closed vowel, the vowel /u/ is a high-back-closed vowel, and the vowel /a/ is an open-central-low vowel. These three vowels, /i, u, a/ are produced at three different positions in the oral cavity and are represented on the vowel diagram. The high vowels /i/ and /u/ have more muscular tension than the low vowel /a/, because the child needs to reach up to phonate the high, closed /i/ and the high, closed /u/ vowels; whereas to phonate the open vowel /a/, the child relaxes his muscular tension and opens his mouth. Both the tongue height and the openness of the oral cavity affect the muscular tension in the production of vowels.

Vowels, Diphthongs, and Consonants

1. **Vowels**—To correspond with the position in the oral cavity, the body movements for the vowels /u, a, i/ are organized at three different points in space. The clinician's body movements for /a/ are made at her waist level. One opens both arms horizontally while phonating /a/, or moves the right arm horizontally from a far-right to far-left position. Both movements represent the same vowel qualities; long duration and less tension. For the vowel /i/, the clinician reaches with both arms in parallel above the waist level and

stretches up on the toes, while vocalizing /i/. For the vowel /u/, the clinician moves both arms to a closed position below the waist while vocalizing /u/. Reaching for the vowels /u/ and /i/ maximizes her muscular tension and differentiates the two tense vowels from the less tense, more relaxed vowel /a/. The other vowel movements are between those two extreme positions in space. On an 11-point scale of perceived tension, the vowel diagram ranges from a relatively low muscular tension of 2 for the less-tense vowel /a/ to a value of 3 for the vowels /i/ and /u/. The mid-high vowels /e/ and /o/ have a mid-value of 2.5 on the scale for perceived tension (Table 2–2).

2. **Diphthongs**—Diphthongs are made with less tension than individual vowels, because diphthongs are coarticulations from an initial vowel position to a second vowel position; for example, /a/ to /ɪ/ in the diphthong /aɪ/. This coarticulation requires less tension to move smoothly from one vowel position to the next. The clinician's body movement for the diphthong /aɪ/ moves from waist level (/a/) to an above-the-head position for /ɪ/. The movement is from the long, open, less tense vowel /a/ to the more tense, closed vowel /ɪ/. In summary, diphthongs require less tension than vowels because of the change in vowel position while coarticulating the two adjacent vowels.

3. **Consonants**—Consonants use more muscular tension than vowels, because the lips are closed more tightly in consonant production. Within the consonants, the voiceless consonants are produced with more muscular tension than the voiced consonants. For example, voiceless, plosive consonants, /p, t, k/ have more tension (level 11 on the scale of perceived tension) than their cognates, /b, d, g/ (level 10). In comparison, the nasal consonant /m/ is longer in duration and less tense than either consonants /p/ or /b/. The shorter duration of /p/ and /b/ create more muscular tension than the longer duration of /m/. The amount of tension is directly affected by the duration of the consonants (Table 2–2).

Body movements for the voiceless consonants /p/ and /t/ are presented above the clinician's waist, similar to the vowel /i/. The /p/ is made with the fingers popping open to simulate the explosion of the consonant /p/. In contrast, the body movement for /t/ is presented above the waist, but with the fingers touching upward to represent the tongue touching the alveolar ridge on the roof of the oral cavity. The place of articulation within the oral cavity is an influential factor in selecting an appropriate body movement.

Table 2–2. A Continuum of Tension for English Phonemes (consonants, vowels and diphthongs) Scale Key = 1 (least tense) to 11 (most tense)

Consonants

Scale	Consonants	Description based on Speech Production
11 (most tense)	/p, t, k/	voiceless plosives
10	/b, d, g/	voiced plosives
9	/tʃ/	voiceless affricative
8	/dʒ/	voiced affricative
7	/f, s, ʃ, h, θ/	voiceless fricatives
6	/v, z, ʒ/	voiced fricatives
5	/w, j/	glides
4	/m, n, ŋ/	nasals
3	/l, r/	laterals

Vowels and Diphthongs

Scale Values	Vowels		Description
3	i	u	High tongue position
	ɪ	ʊ	and Closed
	e	o	
	ɛ	ɚ	
		ə	
2		ɔ	Low tongue position
	ɑ		and Open

Diphthongs

	eɪ	oʊ	High tongue position and Closed
1 (least tense)		ɔɪ	
		ɑɪ	Low tongue position
		ɑʊ	and Open

The clinician's movements for both /b/ and /d/ are made below the waist and with less tension. The clinician rolls his or her hands outward for /b/ (e.g., /bababa/), whereas the clinician uses a downward, more tense movement with closed fists for /d/ (e.g., pounding on the floor or on the knee for /dʌdʌdʌ/).

The clinician's movements for the back consonants /k/ and /g/ are made with elbows moving backward from a midbody position. For /k/, the backward movement is quick and very tense, whereas the backward movement for /g/ is slower and less tense. As previously discussed, the voiceless cognate is produced with more tension than its voiced counterpart.

Coarticulation Movements

For the coarticulation of sounds, the clinician begins with consonants and vowels that are similar in tension; for example, the consonant /m/ and the vowel /a/ have similar tension. The movement for the syllable /ma/ or the syllable /am/ are made at waist level. The syllable /am/ begins with a long /a/ followed by a long /m/ and a falling intonation pattern. The transition from /a/ to /m/ is gradual and the entire movement is made with a very low level of tension. For the syllable /ma/, the movement is slightly more tense, with an upward intonation pattern, but the coarticulation can be made with less tension if the /m/ has a longer duration, less lip contact, and a flat intonation pattern before the transition to the /a/. This is identified as a light articulatory contact in the oral cavity.

Another strategy for changing tension is the use of isometric movements. For example, the clinician creates more muscular tension if she pushes both hands together or pushes the hands against a wall while phonating the more tense vowel /i/ or the more tense consonant /s/. With a longer duration, tension can build over time, and the clinician releases the tension quickly by removing her hands. The changes in isometric tension are useful for keeping a variety of movements for each phoneme. The goal is to have the child feel the changes in tension in his or her body and not concentrate on the visual cues from the clinician's face or specific body movements.

Vibrotactile Speech Input

Although vibrotactile speech input was explained earlier, this section is a review of this treatment tool. The vibrotactile speech input helps the child feel the natural rhythm of speech patterns by sitting on a sounding board and/or wearing a speech wrist vibrator. The sounding board is most effective with infants and toddlers. The infant lies on the board, whereas a toddler can sit on the board. The speech vibrators under the board amplify the speech vibration so the infant or toddler can feel the speech vibrations throughout the entire body. The feeling of the speech vibration helps the young child to feel and imitate the same rhythm and intonation patterns that the clinician produces. For example, the pattern /bʌbʌbʌbʌ (pause) baa/ is felt throughout the young child's body as he or she imitates the clinician's vocal pattern. Wrist speech vibrators can be used with the sounding board or with a child sitting or standing without the vibrating board.

The vibration changes of the intonation patterns help the young child to imitate rising and falling intonation patterns. These changes in intonation patterns help the young child develop intelligible speech patterns and a normal voice quality. Normal voice quality is necessary for improving the child's speech intelligibility.

The vibrotactile speech input is created by the clinician using the Verbotonal Auditory Training Unit. The clinician speaks directly into a high-quality microphone that amplifies speech patterns and transmits the rhythmic pattern to the speech vibrator under the sounding board or on the child's wrist.

Modification of Body Movements with Speech

The clinician begins with a basic speech rhythm of many-to-one, for example, /mamamama (pause) ma/. The goal is to teach the child a basic speech rhythm using a pause and one controlled syllable at the end. If the child imitates the basic rhythm correctly, but substitutes the /b/ for /m/, the clinician accepts his response, because the main goal is to have him feel and imitate the basic speech rhythm. For the many-to-one speech rhythm, the clinician uses an arm movement at waist level in harmony with the rate of a series of syllables (/mamamama/). Then, she stops her movement during her vocal pause, and uses a short movement for the single syllable (/ma/).

For the tension parameter, the clinician first observes the child's overall muscle tone; is the child very tense, very relaxed, or normal? If the child is very tense his error will be the substitution of a more tense phoneme for a less tense phoneme. For example, if the clinician says the target /mama/, the child will say /baba/ or /papa/, because his overall tension facilitates a more tense vocal production. To reduce his tension, the clinician changes her model using the less tense syllable /am/, with a less tense body movement. The longer duration for both /a/ and /m/ for a very gradual coarticulation of the syllable /am/ also helps to reduce tension. With this decrease in tension, the child will be able to produce the target /am/ correctly. When the child is able to imitate the target tension correctly, the clinician changes the target from /am/ to /ma/. If the child sustains low muscular tension, he will imitate the new model /ma/ correctly. Then the clinician reintroduces the original target /mama/, and the child will imitate correctly. Because the child is more involved and aware of body movements, his speech movements are corrected indirectly.

The clinician always begins with whole body movements. For example, she presents a many-to-one speech rhythm by taking a series of slow steps in harmony with the timing of many syllables of /mama-mama/, followed by a whole-body pause, and then one slow step for the single syllable /ma/. Using whole body movements and using arm movements serve the same purpose: to develop basic rhythm patterns, using appropriate duration, rate, and tension.

Once the child's production of basic speech rhythms is stable and consistent, the clinician selects other rhythm patterns for correction. She uses both body movement and speech modification to restimulate the child. This speech modification requires an analysis of the child's error and the appropriate adjustments to the clinician's speech model and body movements. When the child imitates her model correctly, the clinician knows that she provided an optimum stimulation. In short, the child's response indicates whether the clinician provided the child's optimal learning condition. Other treatment tools (e.g., speech vibrator with a low-pass filter) are often added to highlight the clinician's modifications to correct the child's error. These techniques are considered indirect correction. Later, when the child has a stable speech pattern with the correct use of rhythm, intonation, and voice quality patterns, the clinician can use direct correction, in which she gently explains to the child his specific error(s).

Establish Normal Voice Quality

Vibrotactile feedback through the speech vibrator is an effective tool for developing normal voice quality in each young child. The speech vibrator is combined with body movements to create changes in the child's proprioceptive memory and feedback patterns. The combination of movements and speech vibrations helps the child imitate a wide range of intonation patterns; for example, an upward intonation pattern of one octave (e.g., 250 to 500 Hz) or a falling intonation pattern (e.g., 400 to 200 Hz). These wide ranges of intonation patterns improve the child's voice quality, which in turn improves his overall intelligibility.

The speech vibrators and coordinated body movements are also effective for developing a variety of normal vowel productions. In the beginning, most children with hearing impairments vocalize only one or two low vowels (/a/ or /ʌ/). Changing the muscle tension of the body movements and providing vibratory speech input teaches the young child "to reach" for the greater muscular tension of the high vowels, /i/ and /u/. Reaching and stabilizing these high vowels expands the young child's vocal patterns, which improves his voice quality as well as his rhythm and intonation patterns.

Error Analysis and Correction

The Verbotonal Approach requires error analysis and correction at all stages of the young child's development. The Vestibular Strategy of the Verbotonal Approach is targeted in the beginning to develop normal proprioceptive feedback and proprioceptive memory. For example, the child may increase in intonation only slightly (250 to 260 Hz) in response to a body movement simulating rising intonation for the vowel /a/. This change is too small and is perceived as a flat, monotone intonation pattern. Following an error analysis, the clinician modifies her next intonation pattern by using a sweeping body movement to represent her intonation change (250 to 500 Hz). With the aid of the speech vibrator, the child will perceive a greater change through his vestibular system and respond with a greater change (250 to 350 Hz). Next, the clinician adds a more emotional expression in her phonation of the vowel /a/. The young child will then imitate the clinician's intonation change (250 to 500 Hz). Little by little, the child expands his intonation range while receiving feedback from the speech vibrator and the successful body movements. A wider range in muscular tension, facilitated by the body movements, also allows him to develop a wider intonational range. These changes are required for good speech intelligibility. The Vestibular Strategy of error analysis and correction follows the same principles as those of the Auditory and Speech Strategies within the Verbotonal Approach.

Movements Throughout the School Day: Group and Individual Sessions

The clinician begins each school day with one to two hours of movement stimulation and indirect correction along with targeting listening skills. She uses the same language theme throughout the day, keeping movements and listening as part of its stimulation. For example, while in a prereading table activity, she uses body movements and listening for each child as needed. Even on the way to the bathroom or in the lunch room, she consistently incorporates body movements and listening. The goal is to develop listening skills and speech skills throughout the entire school day.

As the children's listening and speaking skills improve, body movements are used less and less. The clinician transitions to a higher level of questions, answers, and discussions, rather than direct imitation. The body movements are used as a treatment tool to provide the optimal learning condition; later, they are used less as the child progresses.

The body movements are most effective as a treatment tool when presented to a group of eight young children who have similar motoric skills. The clinician has the children "work together as a team." The clinician presents a friendly and cooperative environment, which entices each child to want to be a part of the group. Sometimes the clinician uses the child with the "best" performance to demonstrate the correct movement and speech patterns to the other children. The group session usually begins with preschoolers, who first act only as individuals. The children quickly learn to participate as part of a team. Then, the children all move in harmony with the clinician and receive positive feedback from the group. It is a pleasant experience for the children to be supported by and work with their peers in a group.

The individual body movement sessions are the same as the group sessions, except that they are based on the level of the individual child. For infants and toddlers, individual body movements are used in the beginning to prepare the toddler to be a cooperative team member. However, it is more difficult for the clinician to hold the attention of a single child. In most cases, group instruction is more useful. The group sessions require the clinician to be an active listener to each child's imitation; some may be correct, while others may be incorrect. The clinician needs to be a skilled listener and needs to be skillful in selecting the most appropriate speech modifications to correct the errors that are produced.

Movements with Speech Rhymes

Body movements are also used to expand the child's proprioceptive and auditory memory of speech rhymes. The goal is to develop a 3-second memory span of 15 syllables, with a normal speech rate.

The child's memory can be expanded by using speech rhymes that are easy to understand, imitate, retain, and are fun for the child. The clinician can use published nursery rhymes, such as "Humpty Dumpty," "Twinkle, Twinkle," and so forth., or she can make up her own to expand the child's memory pattern for a new phoneme. Her own rhymes range in difficulty from preword syllables to complex words and language. They also range from low tonality phonemes (e.g., /b/) to high tonality consonants (e.g., /s/).

Here are two examples of 4-line speech rhymes:

Example 1

Ah Boo	(2)
Ba Boo	(2)
Boo Boo	(2)
Bah!	(1)
Total	= 7 Syllables

Example 2

Shower Shower	(4)
Take a Shower	(4)
Wash your shoulders	(4)
Take a Shower	(4)
Total	= 16 Syllables

Example 1 uses preword syllables with low tonality. There are a total of seven syllables; two syllables for the first three lines, and one syllable for the fourth line. The rhyme ends with a pause that is a rhythmic "beat." This 7-syllable rhyme is spoken within 1.5 seconds, including the pause.

Example 2 is a 16-syllable rhyme, with 11 words. It is typically spoken in 3.2 seconds. This rhyme is more complex, because it has a high tonality consonant /s/ and has two-syllable words with the syllable stress on the first syllables (e.g., shower and shoulder). The high tonality consonant /s/ is combined with low and mid-tonality vowels. This rhyme also focuses on the consonant /ʃ/ in a weak final position for the word "wash." Both speech rhyme examples are based on a regular rhythmic pattern, with two beats per line. The clinician uses body movements with these speech rhymes in a general way, similar to how a musical conductor would direct a group of singers. She uses flowing body movements to emphasize the two beats per line and to begin and end the speech rhyme.

Auditory Memory

With the Vestibular Strategy, the children imitate the body movements and vocal patterns of the clinician. This imitation helps them to expand their proprioceptive and auditory memory patterns. As the child's auditory memory expands, the clinician requests that the children say the rhyme from memory instead of using direct imitation. As the children's auditory memory expands and develops, the clinician introduces standard universal rhymes and gradually the children are able to recall 3 to 10 rhymes, and they can reproduce them on request. Eventually, the body movements are no longer needed, and the child can learn a new rhyme without any assistance and reproduce it from auditory memory.

The Verbotonal Approach, specifically the Vestibular Strategy, maximizes multisensory speech input. The child's spoken language begins with the basic speech patterns in harmony with nonverbal aspects of language. The child begins with his whole body, and later "hears" with the assistance of his body perception. Production of normal rhythm and intonation patterns helps his voice quality and speech intelligibility. His listening skills also improve. For example, a toddler with normal voice quality will have good speech intelligibility, even though he may only articulate a small percentage of his speech sounds correctly. As another example, an adult with a heavy accent (abnormal rhythm) will likely have poor speech intelligibility. To improve intelligibility, he has to change his speech accent patterns to correspond with the speech patterns of his listeners. This is why rhythm and intonation patterns are emphasized early to infants and toddlers, they are the foundation for both good spoken language skills and good listening skills.

Nonverbal body language is presented in harmony with spoken language. The body language provides visual information to a listener, who shares the same body language. Body language differs between cultures; it is based on their cultural patterns. For example, Italian speakers use different body language than Japanese speakers.

Body movements as a treatment tool function differently than body language. It is critical that the clinician not use one movement as a visual sign or symbol for each of the 43 phonemes. This would be confusing for the child and impossible to remember. The clinician emphasizes the quality of the parameter (parameter-based) or phoneme (phoneme-based) and varies her movements so it is not a sign language.

References

Aras, G. (2000). Hearing in space perception integration. *Proceedings of Verbotonal Symposium.* Zagreb, Croatia: Poliklinka SUVAG.

Aras, G., & Asp, C. (2005). Personal communication.

Asp, C. W. (1985). The Verbotonal method for management of young hearing impaired children. *Ear and Hearing, 6*(1), 39–42.

Asp, C. W., & Guberina, P. (1981). *Verbotonal method for rehabilitating people with communication problems.* New York: NY: World Rehabilitation Fund, Inc.

Ayres, A. J. (1978). Learning disabilities and the vestibular system. *Journal of Learning Disabilities, 11,* 18–29.

Fisher, A. G., Murray, E. A., & Bundy, A. C. (1991). *Sensory integration.* Philadelphia, PA: F.A. Davis Publishing.

Guberina, P. (1972). *The correlation between sensitivity of the vestibular system, and hearing and speech in verbotonal rehabilitation* (Appendix 6, pp. 256–260). Washington, DC: Office of Vocational Rehabilitation, Department of Health, Education, and Welfare.

Horak, F. B., Shumway-Cook, A., Crowe, T. K., & Black, F. O. (1988). Vestibular function and motor proficiency of children with impaired hearing or with learning disability and motor impairments. *Developmental Medicine and Child Neurology, 30*(1), 64–79.

Palmer, L. L. (1999). *Stimulating maturity through accelerated readiness training (SMART).* Minneapolis, MN: Minnesota Learning Resource Center.

Pansini, M. (2000). Verbotonal contribution to audiology and vestibulology. *Proceedings of Verbotonal Symposium.* Zagreb, Croatia: Poliklinka SUVAG.

Sussman, K. D. (1996). *Speech power through rhythmic phonetics* [Video recording]. Redwood City, CA: Jean Weingarten Peninsula Oral School for the Deaf.

CHAPTER

3

Auditory Strategy: Listening Skills for Self-Correction

Once speech pattern recognition is stabilized, listening skills become the dominant modality in a child's speech dialogue. Auditory dominance is perceptually based according to the low-to-high tonotopical organization from the cochlea(s) to the brain. This organization allows the child's brain to select the unique frequency zone (tonality) for each phoneme. For example, the vowels /u-a-i/ and the consonants /m-t-s/ are organized from low-to-high frequency zones. These frequency zones are critical to the child's auditory perception of all 43 vowels, diphthongs, and consonants of the English language. Targeting the phonemes within their perceptual zones is useful in developing an effective treatment plan based on the child's speech errors.

For assessment, the Tonality Word Test (Asp, 1999; Asp & Plyer, 1999) is presented without visual cues to evaluate the child's auditory speech perception in the low, mid, and high frequency zones; for example, "room, cat, cease," respectively. If necessary, the Tonality Syllable Test (/mumu, lala, sisi/) or the Tonality Sentence Test ("Pull the Puppy Up, Tell Tom to Come, Sally Is Sweet") can be administered in conjunction with the Tonality Word Test. Five test items are presented within each tonality zone. The child's performance (percent correct) along with the clinician's error analysis provides information on the child's listening skills in each of the frequency zones. This follows the tonotopic organization of the child's auditory system.

The tonality assessments help the clinician establish the child's optimal listening condition using the Verbotonal Auditory Training Unit (Figure 3–1). The clinician uses the unit's microphone to amplify her speech model and speech modifications. She also allows the child to speak into the microphone so that he can hear his own production amplified. The optimum position of the microphone ensures a quiet signal-to-noise (S/N) ratio of 30 dB. The unit is equipped with a binaural headset and wrist vibrator for each child, so that he can receive both auditory and vibrotactile feedback simultaneously. To highlight the clinician's speech model, one channel of the unit has high-quality, wide-band electrical frequency response (2 to 20,0000 Hz), while the other four channels have filters with precise cutoff frequencies (e.g., 0.25, 0.5, 1, 2, 4, 8 kHz) and slopes (e.g., 0, 6, 12, 20, and 60 dB/octave). This setup allows the clinician to set the optimal frequency zone for each stage of the child's auditory development. The filters are used to

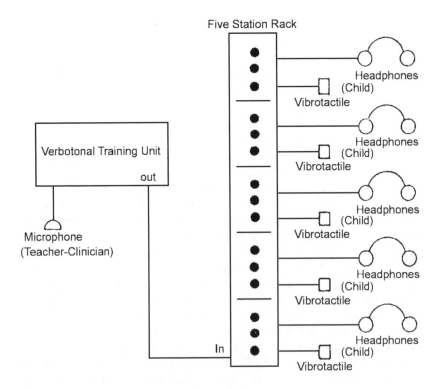

Figure 3–1. Diagram of Verbotonal Training Unit with Children and a Clinician

highlight the target phoneme, while reducing the child's perceptual errors. For example, with a child who has good residual hearing and substitutes an "sh" phoneme for an "s" phoneme, the 6 kHz high-pass filter highlights the "s" in the word "see," and reduces the perception and production of the "sh" error. After the child perceives and produces the "s" correctly, the high-pass filter is removed to facilitate carryover to the wider frequency response of the unit and his hearing aid. At this point, the child's listening skills become dominant for monitoring, controlling, and self-correcting his speech patterns. These refined auditory skills allow the child to successfully understand and communicate with others with reduced visual cues.

The Verbotonal Auditory Training Unit is used in both group and individual treatment sessions in clinic-based and school-based programs (Figure 3–1). With young children, the unit is used for most of the school day to help the child experience consistent high-quality listening. As previously mentioned, the clinician begins by presenting her speech model through the child's binaural headset in a quiet (30 dB S/N), optimal listening condition. When the child has mastered the quiet condition, the training unit is adjusted to add some noise (e.g., 5, 10, or 15 dB S/N) and reverberation (e.g. 0.6, 1.0, or 1.5 second delay) to gradually simulate the adverse listening conditions found in most everyday classrooms and environments.

The child's digital hearing aids are also set to follow his optimal frequency response, which is established by the filter channels that emphasize his residual hearing. This allows a positive transfer from the training unit to his hearing aid(s). For a child with a cochlear implant, a monaural headset can be placed over the contralateral ear to create the condition of binaural speech input. This prepares the child for binaural listening, with a personal hearing aid on one ear and an implant on the other ear. It is important that a binaural listening condition be established at a young age so the child develops accurate auditory perception simultaneously through both systems (hearing aid and cochlear implant).

The clinician uses distance practice as another treatment tool to develop the child's auditory perception in space. Short distances from the unaided ear are used first; for example, 3 to 6 to 9 inches. The child is asked to perceive and repeat familiar words and/or phrases at each of these distances. Later, the child completes distance practice using his hearing aid(s) and/or cochlear implant. The clinician uses distance variation as a treatment tool to stretch the child's aided or implant distance from 3 to 15 feet while maintaining a high level of performance, for example, 90% correct. This practice approximates the listening environment of his classroom and everyday environments.

Auditory Perception: An Overview

The clinician simultaneously stimulates and corrects both speech perception and speech production. He or she works from the easiest perceptual condition up to the most difficult condition. The easiest condition usually includes all possible sensory modalities. The clinician speaks to the child through the Verbotonal Auditory Training Unit, complete with a wrist vibrator and headphones, to provide auditory, tactile, and visual cues of the speech pattern. This multisensory speech input is used in the beginning as an easier condition, but is gradually transferred to auditory-only input, because the goal is to improve the child's auditory perception so that only auditory cues are needed to understand the clinician. Visual cues from facial expressions and body movements are gradually reduced so that the child relies more on the auditory cues. The clinician "trains" the child's brain to perceive the speech signal auditorally even though the acoustic signal is restricted by the peripheral hearing loss. The Verbotonal Approach assumes that the child's brain will compensate for this restricted auditory signal and develop perception for effective communication. This compensation is described as auditory brain transfer.

With the Verbotonal Approach, auditory perception is not viewed from a pure-tone audiogram, which only represents the peripheral hearing loss through the cochlea. From this perspective, if the child's average pure-tone thresholds are 80 or 90 dB HTL, it is often assumed that the child's speech perception cannot be developed. This assumption is based on the classic speech frequencies (500, 1000, 2000 Hz) and does not recognize the child's low-frequency residual hearing below 500 Hz. This assumption also does not account for auditory brain transfer. In contrast, the Verbotonal Approach assumes that the child's brain can be trained to compensate by maximizing his low-frequency residual hearing. If the child is not brain damaged, then the clinician assumes that the child or adult is able to develop auditory speech perception through his residual (low-frequency) hearing if the optimum learning condition is provided. The key to successfully establishing auditory perception is a competent clinician who implements a good strategy and understands the potential of brain perception.

The Ear and the Articulators

Based on the frequencies (pitch) of speech, the tonotopic organization from the child's cochleas to the brain allows the efficient processing, control, and self-correction of his or her speech patterns. Articulatory movements are developmentally linked to the brain's monitoring and control of speech, so they also affect auditory perception. The link between his articulators and his ears helps the child monitor his speech and anticipate the speech rhythm of others for accurate "on-line" speech processing. This is important for the development of normal speech patterns and normal listening skills.

In second language learning, the rhythm, intonation, and phoneme patterns of the native language interfere with the auditory processing of the second language. This is especially true of a person with a heavy foreign accent pattern in the second language, which developed from the motor patterns of the native language. This heavy accent affects his ability to understand others in the second language. This becomes even more apparent in adverse listening conditions with the additional interference of reverberation and noise. A heavy speech accent also negatively affects speech intelligibility, listening skills, and written language. In short, all areas of oral communication are affected by different speech accent patterns.

Anticipation of Speech Rhythms

In a face-to-face dialogue, the listener anticipates the speech rhythms (accent patterns) of the speaker in order to have "on-line" speech processing. The typical speaker produces up to 15 phonemes per second. This rapid articulation of phonemes becomes a perceptual blur if the speech rhythms are not anticipated. For example, foreign language listeners cannot accurately anticipate the speech rhythms of a native language user, because the foreign and native languages have different patterns of speech rhythms. The foreign language listener has difficulty distinguishing where one word ends and the next begins.

Anticipation of speech rhythms is a developmental milestone with infants and toddlers; it is learned naturally in a preword "speech dialogue" between the mother and her infant. The mother responds vocally to her infant, establishing the articulator-to-ear link, which is the basis of the infant's functional brain processing of speech patterns.

The articulator-to-ear link is critical to providing treatment for speech and/or language disorders. If the infant-toddler only responds by pointing or selecting the correct word in a picture, his articulator-to-ear link is not developing. Without this link, anticipation of speech rhythms will be limited.

Tonotopic Organization: Cochlea to the Brain

The left and right cochleas are tonotopically organized with 30,000 receptors between them and the auditory-processing part of the brain. The auditory range of frequencies (pitch perception) is from 20 Hz to 20,000 Hz. Within the cochlea, the low frequencies (20–200 Hz) are processed in the upper one-third of the cochlea, the medium frequencies (200–2000 Hz) are processed in the middle one-third of the cochlea, and the high frequencies (2000–20,000 Hz) are processed in the lower one-third of the cochlea. In short, tonotopic receptors are "lows" at 100 Hz, "mids" at 1000 Hz, and "highs" at 10,000 Hz. The central nervous system (from the cochlear nuclei to the primary auditory cortex) is tuned to these frequencies by a place code (tonotopic) and a rate code (speed). The cochlea is also sensitive to different intensities, with the lower and higher frequency zones requiring more physical intensity (dB) than the midfrequency zone to establish speech detection and equal loudness thresholds.

Tonotopic organization allows the brain to discriminate among the 43 different phonemes that comprise spoken language. These phonemes have 43 different frequency responses that provide spectral pitch cues to perceiving them differently. For example, the vowel /a/ and the vowel /i/ have very different frequency responses; therefore the spectral pitch difference is clear and it is easy for the brain to perceive the difference. The vowels /i/ and /ɪ/ are closer in frequency responses, so the listener has to concentrate to perceive the spectral pitch difference. Similarly, consonants /b/ and /s/ have a large and easily perceived spectral pitch difference, whereas /s/ and /ʃ/ have similar frequency responses making the perception of their spectral pitch difference less salient.

The Verbotonal Approach uses the tonotopical organization to explain how the child's brain is "tuned" for the identification of each phoneme. The tonality zones (low-mid-high) correspond to the tonotopic organization in the brain for monosyllabic words, such as "moo" (low), "cat" (mid), and "see" (high). The tonality zones highlight the difference among phonemes; the phonemes are organized within these zones rather than being randomized across a wide frequency response.

The Brain's Bandwidth for Speech Processing

The brain has an extended low-frequency bandwidth that is tonotopically sensitive to the speech frequencies (pitches) from 2 Hz to 20,000 Hz. The extended low speech frequencies can be transmitted with a vibrotactile wrist vibrator from the Verbotonal Auditory Training Unit.

The vibrotactile range is 2 Hz to 1000 Hz. This range includes vestibular-cochlear hearing, which helps to establish the link between the articulators and the ear.

The speech spectrum (frequency range) of normal conversational speech extends over the entire bandwidth of the brain. Because of the dynamic nature of conversational speech, the vocal patterns have up to 5 syllables per second and up to 15 phonemes per second. The quick articulatory changes (coarticulation) spread the speech energy across the entire bandwidth. As an analogy, a continuous pure-tone test frequency of 1000 Hz only has acoustic energy at 1000 Hz; however, when it is interrupted at a rapid rate, the energy spreads outside the 1000 Hz center frequency. The same principle applies to a sustained vowel versus an interrupted vowel production. Interrupted vowels occur in conversational speech at a rate of five syllables per second. Other features of sound production also extend the acoustic spectrum. For example, the consonant /p/ has a breathy release of air (aspiration) that has a wide acoustic spectrum extending below 100 Hz. Rhythm and intonation patterns can be perceived below 125 Hz, and they are perceived with an accuracy similar to using a wide bandwidth (Kim & Asp, 2002). Such low frequencies are optimal for pattern perception.

Differences in the Brain's Bandwidth: Child Versus Adult

The child with normal hearing develops his auditory perception using the entire wide bandwidth of his brain. An infant begins to develop his perception by first "feeling" his mother's speech rhythms as she holds him closely, similar to when he was a fetus. An infant or toddler with a severe speech communication disorder needs similar experiences and access to a wide bandwidth.

To simulate these important vibrotactile experiences, the treatment strategy of the Verbotonal Approach begins at the preword level with speech modification and speech rhythms presented through the headsets, body movements, and vibrotactile speech input through the Verbotonal Auditory Training Unit. The child develops by feeling the speech rhythms. This is called the "Mommy-Baby Method" (Guberina, 1972). This method provides the child with emotional security and motivates him to interact with his clinician as he does with his mother.

Normal adults who speak the same native language can easily engage in a normal speech dialogue by listening over the narrow, three-octave bandwidth of a telephone (300 to 3000 Hz). They are able to do this because of their advanced auditory perception and accurate antic-

ipation of speech rhythms, plus they have internalized all the proprioceptive speech rhythm patterns. A narrow bandwidth is sufficient for a
telephone conversation or understanding speech through a television or
radio. The normal adult's brain compensates by "filling in" the missing
frequencies. This is accomplished by auditory brain speech transfer. For
an adult with a heavy foreign accent, the narrow bandwidth of the telephone is not always sufficient. These individuals prefer a face-to-face
dialogue with a wide bandwidth and the visual cues of body language.

In diagnostic audiology, this narrow bandwidth (300 to 3000 Hz) is
called the "conversational speech zone." Acoustic information for 80%
of the phonemes are included in this narrow frequency range. In fact,
most hearing aids and cochlear implants are set for an even narrower
bandwidth, such as 500 to 2000 Hz. This strategy of amplifying only a
narrow frequency range is based on the adult model for listening over
the telephone and also to avoid masking by the low-frequency ambient
noise (below 500 Hz).

The normal adult brain is capable of accurately perceiving conversational speech even when the "conversational speech zone" is not
available. For example, when conversational speech is passed through
a 300 Hz low-pass filter and a 3000 Hz high-pass filter simultaneously,
it is fully understood by the listener. Bimodal speech perception combines two different bandwidths. Each of these bandwidths has 0%
understanding by itself. For example, the 300 Hz low-pass filter and
the 3,000 Hz high-pass filter each have 0% intelligibility for conversational speech. When both bandwidths are presented simultaneously,
however, there is a full bimodal perception of 90%. The low-frequency
rhythm and intonation patterns of conversational speech enhance the
brain's perception of the high frequencies. In other words, the structures
of rhythm and intonation patterns provide a framework for the adult
brain to fill in and perceive the individual phonemes in conversational
speech, even though they were actually filtered out of the signal.

In a separate study, a low-frequency bandwidth (55–110 Hz,
110–220 Hz, or 220–440 Hz) improved speech perception of words
when it was added to the high-frequency bandwidth (1100 to 2200 Hz).
This experiment supports the strategy of the bimodal (discontinuous)
model for the brain's speech perception.

Perceptual Brain Transfer:
Maximize the Residual Hearing

It is important to develop the listening skills of a child or adult with a
hearing loss through his most sensitive residual hearing. This is accomplished through auditory brain transfer, which is the brain's ability to

compensate through neuroplastic development. The high-frequency speech energy is perceived through the low-frequency residual hearing.

The Verbotonal Approach is to develop the low-frequency residual hearing below 1000 Hz. Developing the functional residual hearing of a client with a high-frequency hearing loss by using a 1000 Hz low-pass filter tuned to the client's sensitive region results in 100% listening skills (word recognition) for conversational speech. Perceptual brain transfer, using the best areas of hearing sensitivity (low frequencies) to compensate for the worst areas of hearing sensitivity, offers hope for individuals with mild to profound hearing loss.

In contrast, most conventional strategies amplify the area of the greatest loss (hearing aids) to achieve aided pure-tone detection thresholds below 25 dB HL. For example, an unaided threshold of 90 dB HL at 4000 Hz would have a 70 dB hearing aid gain to achieve an aided threshold of 20 dB HL. Although the threshold levels are reduced, the excessive frequency amplification (gain) of the high frequencies usually results in recruitment, which is an uncomfortable growth in loudness. The high-frequency gain also forces the tonality errors to go toward the high frequencies, for example, /s/ produced for /ʃ/. In short, high-powered amplification can be painful and can result in poor speech perception.

Another example of bimodal (discontinuous) hearing-aid fitting is passing the low-frequency speech rhythms naturally through an open or free-field earmold. A narrow-band, high-frequency hearing aid is then added with a small gain of 5 to 20 dB. This bimodal strategy works effectively when the patient has low-frequency residual hearing that is functional. In short, the low-frequency speech energy is passed naturally, and the high-frequency speech energy is mildly amplified by the high-frequency hearing aid. The client's ear is not occluded by an earmold, so his speech sounds natural to him.

Dead Frequency Zones

Recent research has demonstrated that high-frequency pure-tone thresholds greater than 70 dB HL may be dead frequency zones and may not be useful for high-frequency speech perception. When this situation occurs, mirroring the hearing loss by amplifying these "dead" frequency zones may actually hinder rather than help the client's speech recognition.

In 1968, Bredberg reported hair cell damage in the human cochlea of an individual with hearing loss through postmortem examination. The hair cell damage appeared in the right cochlea of a 71-year-old man who worked in a high intensity, noisy sawmill for many years. His pure-tone audiogram for his right ear shows normal hearing (0–25 dB) for up to 500 Hz, and a mild (30 dB) to severe (70 dB) hearing loss above 1000 Hz. A 70 dB hearing loss "notch" at 2000 Hz is typical in noise-induced hearing loss. The question is: "Does the 70 dB loss at 2000 Hz represent a dead frequency zone?" Through physical examination, the right cochlea shows an almost complete degeneration of radial nerves in the osseus spiral lamina as well as a corresponding degeneration of the organ of Corti in the region between 135° and 270° of the cochlea. A few inner hair cells are present, but all outer hair cells have degenerated. Bredberg's (1968) analysis suggests that the 70 dB HL pure-tone threshold at 2000 Hz is a dead zone for both outer and inner hairs.

For Bredberg's (1968) client, the optimal frequency response (OFR) would be a 1000 Hz low-pass filter and a 6000 Hz high-pass filter to present the speech signal. This allows the 2000 Hz dead zone to be avoided.

Modifications of Basic Audiometry

After receiving appropriate medical clearance, standard pure-tone thresholds and speech audiometry are completed on all patients. The test frequencies for pure-tone thresholds are 125 to 8000 Hz for most audiometers. For the Verbotonal Approach, the extended low-frequency thresholds of 125 Hz and 250 Hz and the extended high-frequency thresholds of 6000 Hz and 8000 Hz are needed to identify the more sensitive areas of the residual hearing. In fact, the entire frequency spectrum, including 20 to 125 Hz and 8000 to 20,000 Hz is helpful in determining the bandwidths with the most sensitivity.

For speech audiometry, both speech reception threshold (SRT) and speech detection threshold (SDT) are obtained in each ear. The SRT is the lowest dB level at which the client correctly repeats back 50% of the spondee test words (e.g., baseball, hotdog, etc.); the SDT is the lowest dB level at which the patient detects the presence of the spondee words. The difference (dB) between SRT and SDT helps distinguish if the client's residual hearing is functional. For example, if the client's SRT is 5 dB above his SDT, he needs only 5 dB of amplification to correctly identify 50% of the spondee words. However, if he needs 40 dB above his SDT (e,g., SRT = 95 dB, SDT = 55 dB), his residual hearing is not functional. The Verbotonal Approach will help decrease the client's SRT so he or she can understand the spondee words with reduced loudness (amplification). For example, the 5 dB difference may reduce to a 2 dB difference, and the 40 dB difference to a 15 dB difference. When the client needs less loudness (lower SRT), the sensitive low-frequency zone is considered functional. The client's brain has developed low-frequency perceptual transfer for the high frequencies, and thus requires less amplification. Avoiding excessive amplification, especially in the dead frequency zones, allows the client to function more efficiently in adverse, noisy situations.

The Client's SRT and Bandwidth

An SRT "fold-over" technique is used to determine optimal bandwidth or optimal frequency zone for amplification. This is accomplished by folding the bottom edge of the pure-tone audiogram at the exact level of the client's SRT plotted threshold levels. For example, if the client is able to repeat 50% of the spondee words correctly at a bandwidth of 125 to 1000 Hz, then this frequency range is the optimal bandwidth (optimal frequency zone) that should be amplified with a hearing aid or the Verbotonal Auditory Training Unit. The client's optimal bandwidth is important for successful speech processing, because it minimizes perceptual distortion from the area of the greatest hearing loss. It can be assumed that the hearing in the low frequencies is probably contributing most to understanding speech; this supports the idea of folding the audiogram to the SRT dB level. If the SRT corresponds best with the pure tone average (PTA) of the lower frequencies, then functional residual hearing is most likely centered around the lower frequencies. This technique ensures that the area of greatest loss is not amplified, therefore, minimizing distortion.

Optimal Frequency Response (OFR)

To determine optimal frequency response (OFR), which is the frequency range at which the client's speech perception is the greatest, the Verbotonal Auditory Training Unit can filter out the areas of the greatest hearing loss and pass only the speech frequencies through the client's most sensitive residual hearing. The optimal frequency response (OFR) is developed by the clinician through a series of treatment sessions with the headphones and vibrotactile speech input of the training unit. Five parallel channels are used. These are wideband, low-pass, low-peaking, high-pass, and high-peaking filters. This will be explained in more detail later in the text.

The first task is to set the low-pass filter to match the client's pure-tone thresholds below 1000 Hz. For example, the first OFR would be a 1000 Hz low-pass filter set with a 0 dB slope toward low frequencies and a 20 dB slope toward high frequencies. The clinician checks the child's auditory perception through the low-pass filter using the Tonality Word Test. Depending on the test results, the clinician adjusts the low-pass filter in slopes and cutoff frequencies to improve the client's perception. Then the clinician adds a high-pass filter, which usually adds 20% or more to speech reception when paired with the low-pass filter. The speech vibrator is added as needed.

Unaided Distance: Using the Fletcher Graph

"Unaided distance" is the distance in feet or meters between the client's ears and clinician's mouth with no amplification used. Unaided distance is measured in a regular therapy room without any special acoustic treatment.

To estimate the client's unaided distance, the Fletcher Distance Graph was constructed (Guberina, 1972). The graph is based on the precise speech measurement made by Harvey Fletcher, a scientist at Bell Telephone Labs. Table 3–1 displays the graph with the horizontal axis as the low-to-high tonalities and the vertical axis as the estimated distance (feet or meters) needed to achieve a most comfortable loudness level (MCL). The vertical column in the graph's center is the client's speech reception threshold (dB HTL). To estimate the distance for a client with an average pure-tone threshold of 92 dB, the clinician's mouth needs to be half an inch from the client's ear. At this distance, the clinician presents the tonality test words. Then, the client repeats what he or she "hears," and is instructed not to guess. This is a measurement of perception, so guessing would interfere with the results. This ½-inch distance is considered the closest and loudest speech condition possible.

During the unaided test, the clinician always speaks at the same most comfortable loudness level. For example, the clinician does not raise or lower his or her voice during the test condition; only the distance is varied to establish the most comfortable loudness condition.

Table 3–1. Estimation of Unaided Distance Based on Fletcher Distance Graph

3 feet	35 dB	10 meters (33 feet)
40 inches	55 dB	1 meter (3 feet)
4 inches	75 dB	
0.6 inch	92 dB	3.5 cm $\leqq$ 1 inch

Also, the clinician begins with the client's better ear. She instructs the client to plug his or her contralateral ear with an index finger or with an earplug. This minimizes crossover to the nontest ear.

As another example, for a client with an average pure-tone threshold of 66 dB HTL, the clinician uses the Fletcher Graph's unaided distance estimate of 12 inches. The clinician can shorten (6 inches) or lengthen (24 inches) this distance to evaluate if the increase or decrease improves the client's speech recognition. He also asks the client to indicate which distance (6, 12, or 24 inches) is the most comfortable loudness level for speech. Based on this observation and on the client's feedback, she selects the optimum distance for MCL and speech recognition. She then presents the entire Tonality Word Test at this level.

A third client has a 46 dB pure-tone average. The clinician refers to the Fletcher Graph, which indicates an estimated unaided distance of 10 feet. As in the previous example, the clinician decreases (5 feet) and increases (20 feet) the distance to determine the optimum distance for speech recognition and the client's most comfortable loudness level. If the optimum distance is 10 feet, the clinician presents the Tonality Word Test at 10 feet.

In summary, the three estimated distances for the three different clients were ½ inch, 12 inches, and 10 feet, respectively. The Fletcher graph provided a target distance to begin evaluating each of these clients. With the Verbotonal Approach, all clients will improve (increase) their distance for speech recognition with listening therapy. After a 30-minute session on the Verbotonal Auditory Training Unit, the earphones are removed and the client's distance increases.

The low-mid-high syllable test of /mumu/, /lala/, and /sisi/ of the Verbotonal Approach can be used as a quick speech recognition test at the optimal unaided distance. For example, the third client discussed, with a 10-foot optimal unaided distance, may correctly repeat back /mumu/ and /lala/, but he may substitute /ʃiʃi/ for /sisi/. This result suggests that the client has adequate perception of low and mid-frequencies, but the /ʃ/ substitution for the high /s/ speech sounds suggests a lack of good high-frequency perception.

Verbotonal Speech Audiometry

Detection Thresholds with Filtered Speech Syllables

Miner and Danhauer (1977) reported the relationship between the formant frequencies of vowels and the optimal octaves in the perception of vowels presented at a most comfortable loudness level. They reported the optimal octave bandwidths allowed for correct perception and identification of each vowel, and that these octaves are similar to some of the formant frequencies of the vowels that were tested.

Following this optimal octave concept, the filtered speech detection thresholds are obtained with eight nonsense syllables called logotomes. These logotomes are /brubru, mumu, bubu, vovo, lala, keke, shishi, and sisi/. These test items are all homogeneous syllables, where both the consonant and the vowel within the syllable are from similar optimal octaves. For example, /l/ and /a/ in the syllable /la/ both have mid-frequency optimal octaves and /s/ and /i/ in the syllable /si/ both have high-frequency optimal octaves. Each syllable is spoken twice to achieve the natural speech rhythm of a two-syllable utterance.

To determine speech detection threshold (SDT), the tests items are passed through their optimal octave bandwidths. For example, /lala/ is passed through the optimal octave bandwidth with a 1000 Hz center frequency. The SDT is compared to the client's pure-tone threshold at 1000 Hz. Because of the wider bandwidth, the logotome speech detection threshold usually shows better sensitivity than the pure-tone thresholds. For example, the 1000 Hz pure-tone threshold would be 50 dB HL; whereas the 1000 Hz logotome threshold would be 40 dB HL. The speech detection threshold shows better sensitivity; therefore, these thresholds can be used to identify the client's residual hearing, including "islands of hearing" not identified with the pure-tone thresholds.

Low, High, and Bimodal Perceptual Transfer

To test the client's potential for auditory brain transfer (from a high to low frequency), a high-frequency logotome (e.g., /sisi/) is tested through an unoptimal low-frequency octave (e.g., a center frequency of 500 Hz or lower). The optimal and the unoptimal octave thresholds are compared to determine if the brain is more sensitive for /sisi/ through the low- or high-frequency zone. This comparison is also made by passing a low-frequency logotome (e.g., /vovo/) through a high bandwidth (e.g., a center frequency of 2000 Hz and above).

For bimodal transfer (using low and high frequencies together), the logotome /sisi/ is passed simultaneously through the high-frequency optimal octave of 3,000 Hz and a low-frequency octave of 300 Hz. If the bimodal threshold is better than the optimal octave by itself, then the client's brain has the ability to compensate by using both the low and high frequencies together. Additionally, by using a wide bandwidth, detection thresholds are obtained using logotomes without filtering. The three tests of perceptual transfer (optimal, unoptimal, and without filtering) are useful in determining the brain's potential for perceiving speech sounds (phonemes) with restricted bandwidth(s) and for assessing the optimal condition for speech perception for each client.

Tonality Max: Performance Intensity Function (% PI)

The Tonality Test provides a percent correct score (%) for the perception of low-, mid-, and high-tonality zones. This provides information that helps the clinician make appropriate hearing aid and/or cochlear implant adjustments (Asp & Plyler, 1999). The tonality test words are also used to evaluate the client's performance as a function of increased intensity (dB). This is called the performance-intensity (PI) function. The PI function is based on normal-hearing listeners, where 0 dB is the lowest speech detection threshold. At 30 dB above his or her detection threshold, the average normal listener perceives 100% of the test words correctly. Therefore, the Tonality Max is 100% at the 30 dB level for normal-hearing listeners. This is the lowest dB level a normal-hearing person can achieve a maximum score of 100%.

To create the Tonality PI Function for a client, 10 tonality words are presented at each 10-dB interval above the client's speech detection threshold. For example, if the client's detection threshold is 50 dB, then 10 tonality words are presented at each 10-dB step above 50 dB (e.g., 60, 70, 80, 90, and 100 dB). If the maximum tonality score of 100% occurs at 100 dB, then the Tonality Max is 100 dB. This indicates that the client needs 50 dB of amplification to achieve his Tonality Max at 100 dB. His Tonality Max is high (compared to the 30 dB Tonality Max of normal listeners), and his PI Function has a gradual slope.

As a general rule, the steeper the slope of the PI function, the less amplification needed to achieve Tonality Max. In comparison, the PI function for normal listeners is even steeper for spondee words (e.g., baseball, hotdog), because these words are easier to perceive. The listener can guess the word "baseball" if he hears either "base" or "ball." In contrast, nonsense syllables have a more gradual function because the listener is unable to guess; she has to hear both the consonant and the vowel to perceive it correctly (e.g., /ba/, the listener has to hear both /b/ and /a/). The Tonality Max for nonsense syllables occurs at 40 dB or greater for normal-hearing listeners because of the difficulty of the speech items.

Some hearing-impaired clients have "rollover" PI functions, because their performance gets worse as more amplification is added. For example, an 80% score decreases to 50% when amplification is increased by 20 dB (60 dB to 80 dB). This indicates that the client cannot tolerate more amplification, possibly due to recruitment. This information is useful in understanding the client's limitations with amplification.

The 10-word procedure described has three low-, four mid-, and three high-tonality words in each set, covering the three main tonality zones. So, five presentation levels can be evaluated using only 50 of the tonality words. This organization of presentation avoids excessive testing that may fatigue the client. In contrast, with Phonetically-Balanced (PB) Max Testing, the audiologist presents the entire 50 test words at one presentation level (dB). With the same number of test words, the tonality PI function is achieved at 30, 40, 50, 60, and 70 dB. With the use of tonality-grouped words, all three tonality zones can be tested over five different dB levels, while minimizing the client's fatigue. This provides more information for a treatment plan.

The writer of this book prefers using the Tonality Max method because the entire PI function is evaluated, thus avoiding the degree of error that is introduced with estimation. Kaplan, Gladstone, and Lloyd (1993) reported that using one level for estimating PB Max is not the best method. Rather, having more than one sensation level presentation increases the accuracy of the estimate.

Relationship Between Pure-Tone and Speech Audiometry

Puretone detection thresholds are used to document a peripheral hearing loss and to provide information for diagnosis. It is an effective test for establishing the integrity of a peripheral hearing loss. If needed, bone conduction testing is used to identify middle ear problems. When an effective treatment improves the client's performance outcome by 30%, the pure-tone audiogram still shows the same pure-tone thresholds; therefore, pure-tone detection threshold testing is not useful for measuring or predicting performance outcomes.

On the other hand, Verbotonal speech audiometry with optimal logotome detection helps identify "islands of hearing" and can be used to determine the bandwidth of the client's residual hearing. This information helps to establish an effective treatment plan. Tonality testing, using error analysis, also provides useful information for both the level of amplification needed and the adjustment of the frequency response on the hearing aid or Verbotonal Auditory Training Unit. For example, an /f/ substitution for /s/ provides the clinician with direction for changing the frequency response. In this case, adding some high frequencies and/or cutting some low frequencies would move the /f/ error closer to the /s/ target.

In conventional audiology, the phonetically-balanced (PB) word lists are used to compare two hearing aids or two settings on the same hearing aid. The typical PB test procedure encourages the client to guess, rather than repeat exactly what he or she hears. This does not provide a true measure of what the client is able to hear. If two 50-word PB tests have a one-word difference (80% vs. 82%), the 2% difference is too small to be meaningful. An effective error analysis procedure of what the client actually hears would make PB testing more meaningful, but in most cases, error analysis is not used. This has reduced the effectiveness of PB testing for selecting amplification or for evaluating performance outcome.

In short, Verbotonal audiometry, if used correctly, provides useful information for both hearing aid placement and cochlear implants in terms of functional residual hearing (including "islands of hearing"), better treatment plans through a more extensive understanding of what the client is hearing, and performance outcomes in "real-world" situations.

Functional Assessment

Functional assessment includes both suprasegmentals and tonality assessment beyond the test booth. The unaided, aided, and Verbotonal Auditory Training Unit test scores are compared to determine the optimal frequency response (OFR) for each client. Ideally the Verbotonal audiometry assessment is completed before the functional measures. Both types of assessment are important to understand how the client's brain processes speech.

A comprehensive assessment strategy is needed for making an appropriate diagnosis and determining an effective treatment plan. The assessment procedures should be based on the norms of children and adults with normal hearing, normal communication skills, and appropriate age levels. As a point of caution, "overtesting" and "labeling" the client should be avoided, and an evidence-based theoretical model should be followed.

The Verbotonal Approach emphasizes functional assessment that enhances effective treatment. For example, based on residual hearing and/or an error analysis, what are the performance targets of the treatment protocol? Are they realistic and functional? These are questions that functional assessment procedures target.

Assessment with a Treatment Strategy

To obtain reliable and valid measures, it is necessary to control the child's behavior. Sometimes behavior management is difficult, and the caregivers are not always helpful with controlling the behavior. In these cases, the clinician has to be a "master" at developing immediate bonding and control, usually without the mother's presence. "Tough love" sets the tone for a no-nonsense approach, where the child learns what behaviors are acceptable and not acceptable. Establishing this rapport and setting limits takes time; therefore, a series of functional assessments with treatment sessions are needed to obtain reliable and valid information. An error analysis of the child's response to treatment provides critical assessment information and "targets" for future treatment. For example, can the child imitate a basic many-to-one speech rhythm pattern? The child may not achieve this target until the fifth session. Initiating the child's stimulability was not immediate, but still very important in developing a realistic prognosis and treatment plan.

Ideally, a medical-educational model is used for effective assessment and treatment. This model has been developed at the Verbotonal Speech and Hearing Center in Zagreb, Croatia. The medical personnel are required to have treatment experience to better understand the relationship between a functional assessment and an effective treatment.

The clinician develops a close working relationship with the appropriate medical specialists. This relationship is more common now with the increase in cochlear implant surgery. The physician not only provides medical clearance, but also performs surgery. The surgeons are interested in effective treatment to enhance the patient's surgical outcome. This creates opportunities for an effective medical-educational model to be implemented.

Ideally, standard audiometry and vestibular testing should be completed by the client's physician (ENT or pediatrician) and the audiologist to ensure proper medical clearance and to provide basic diagnostic information. Our functional assessment should be compared to this diagnostic information to determine areas of agreement and areas that need further evaluation.

For preschool children, the clinician should be knowledgeable in the standard developmental stages of vocalization, cognition, communication, feeding, phonology, auditory-verbal, mean length of utterance, morphemes, and language. These stages are published under language development and language disorders. Knowledge of these developmental stages is important to relate the child's current development with "normal" development.

Suprasegmental Assessment

With the Verbotonal approach, the first step is to assess the motor skills of the infant or toddler. The clinician can administer some standard motoric tests, but should also consider consulting with a physical therapist and/or occupational therapist for additional assessment information. If motor delays are observed, specific vestibular developmental exercises are implemented. These exercises are explained in detail in chapter 2.

Vibrotactile speech input of the clinician's voice through the Verbotonal Auditory Training Unit is used to determine if the infant or toddler can feel and imitate speech rhythm. The tactile input of the speech rhythm is presented through a vibratory board and/or one or more vibrators attached to the infant or toddler's wrist or ankle. Generally, peripheral vibratory speech input is more successful than central input; however, if there is fluid or infection in the middle ear, the vibrotactile speech input is more effective on the head. This allows the input to bypass the 30-dB conductive hearing loss. In the presence of a conductive hearing loss, medical treatment is needed.

The clinician should observe and note the level of body and/or facial tension associated with stiff or slumpy limbs. Observations should be made on the excessiveness of peripheral (arms and legs) tension and/or central (lips, tongue, etc.) tension. Is there a consistent and clear relationship between the peripheral and central tension? These are all considerations that should be made during the assessment procedures. The infant-toddler's spatial awareness should also be considered. Is the child aware of his or her relationship to others, and can he or she move freely in different directions while coordinating arms, legs, head, and so forth? Does the child have good balance? If the child uses sign language as a means of communication, are his or her signs smooth and meaningful, and can the child vocalize in harmony with his or her signs?

These questions are addressed in the preword suprasegmental assessment, in which an error analysis is completed following a stimulus-response elicitation paradigm. The seven speech parameters of rhythm, intonation, tension, pause, time (duration), pitch, and loudness are evaluated both independently and in conjunction with one another.

First, the clinician evaluates the infant/toddler's initial response to her or her voice. Does the child "feel" the speech rhythm through the vibrotactile speech input? Does he or she hear it through the headsets? What is the child's response to the "on" and "off" of the clinician's voice? Can he or she imitate a basic speech rhythm of many-to-one syllables (e.g., /babababa (pause) ba/)? If the child is able to produce syllables, the other parameters are evaluated.

Some examples of assessment questions of the other parameters include: Can the child perceive and imitate a long syllable duration versus a short syllable duration? Using /ba/ or /da/, can he or she imitate a normal rate of five repetitions per second? Can the child produce syllables at a faster rate (e.g., eight per second) and slower rate (two per second)? When the child changes tempo, can he or she maintain both good voice quality and accurate articulation of the phonemes?

Suprasegmental Tests

The Tennessee Test of Rhythm and Intonation Patterns (T-TRIP) with 25 test items is administered by live or recorded audiotape presentation (Koike & Asp, 1982). The test items range from one to nine syllables, varying in rhythm, tempo, and intonation pattern. The test results are compared to standardized norms of three and five-year-old children (60% and 86% correct, respectively).

Tonality Tests

The Tennessee Tonality Word and Sentence Test (Asp & Plyler, 1999) is administered in low-, mid-, and high-tonality categories (Tables 3–2 and 3–3). Each category has five presentations; for example, a low-tonality word might be "moon" and a low-tonality sentence might be "Pull the Puppy Up." In contrast, a high-tonality word would be "cheese" and a high-tonality sentence would be "Sally Is My Sister." The percent correct in each tonality category, including words and sentences, is computed (e.g., four out of five correct is 80%).   ·

For the Tonality Word Test, the percent correct for the vowels and the consonants are computed separately to provide functional assessment information for treatment. Typically, the percent correct for the vowel score will be similar to the sentence score. If the young child has good rhythm and intonation perception; his word score may be lower than both his vowel score and his sentence score, because of his consonant errors in words (e.g., "hat" for "sat"). The sentence score more accurately predicts how the young child functions in everyday conversation. This is especially true for children with good perception of rhythm and intonation patterns.

Table 3-2. Tonality Test for Word

Conditions: Unaided Distance,   Listen/SUVAG,   Hearing Aids,   Cochlear Implant

Low-Tonality

	Phoneme			
1st	C	V	C	2nd

1. moon / mun /
2. rope / rop /
3. bowl / bol /
4. bone / bon /
5. move / mov /

Low Words = 1st _____ %, 2nd _____ %

Mid-Tonality

	Phoneme			
1st	C	V	C	2nd

1. dad / dæd /
2. hot / hat /
3. duck / dʌk /
4. tag / tæg /
5. tack / tak /

Mid Words = 1st _____ %, 2nd _____ %

High-Tonality

	Phoneme			
1st	C	V	C	2nd

1. fish / fɪʃ /
2. teeth / tiθ /
3. cheese / tʃiz /
4. thief / θif /
5. sit / sɪt /

High Words = 1st _____ %, 2nd _____ %

Total: 1st: _____ %
2nd: _____ %
Total (1st + 2nd): _____ %

Low-Tonality

	Phoneme			
1st	C	V	C	2nd

1. boom / bum /
2. pool / pul /
3. robe / rob /
4. mole / mol /
5. roam / rom /

Low Words = 1st _____ %, 2nd _____ %

Mid-Tonality

	Phoneme			
1st	C	V	C	2nd

1. hat / hæt /
2. rag / ræg /
3. rock / rak /
4. tag / tæg /
5. cut / kʌt /

Mid Words = 1st _____ %, 2nd _____ %

High-Tonality

	Phoneme			
1st	C	V	C	2nd

1. kiss / kɪs /
2. this / ðɪs /
3. cease / sis /
4. chick / tʃɪk /
5. keys / kiz /

High Words = 1st _____ %, 2nd _____ %

Total: 1st: _____ %
2nd: _____ %
Total (1st + 2nd): _____ %

Table 3–3. Tonality Test for Sentence

Testee: _____ Date: _____ Tester: _____

Conditions: Unaided Distance, Listen/SUVAG, Hearing Aids, Cochlear Implant

Test 1

Low-Tonality	No.	Cor.	Mid-Tonality	No.	Cor.	High-Tonality	No.	Cor.
1. Pull the puppy up	4		1. Tell Tom to come	4		1. My feet itch	3	
2. Mama blew a bubble	4		2. Let's drink some coke	4		2. She is my sister	4	
3. Warm up the bread	4		3. We ate dinner	3		3. Tea is cheap	3	
4. No more bubbles	3		4. He wrote a letter	4		4. She saw the show	4	
5. Up goes the boy	4		5. Give me a light	4		5. Is your sister sick?	4	
Subtotal	19	%	Subtotal	19	%	Subtotal	18	%

Test I Overall—Total (56 = 19 + 19 + 18): %

Test II

Low-Tonality	No.	Cor.	Mid-Tonality	No.	Cor.	High-Tonality	No.	Cor.
1. Blow up the ball	4		1. Tell the cook it's good	4		1. My sister's sick	3	
2. No don't do that	4		2. He hit his lip	4		2. Show Sally your socks	4	
3. Buy mama an apple	4		3. Let's play house	4		3. She saw zebras	3	
4. Blow bubbles at me	4		4. Mail the letter today	4		4. It's easy to seesaw	4	
5. Mama made the puppy	4		5. Tell Linda hello	3		5. Sally is sweet	3	
Subtotal	20	%	Subtotal	18	%	Subtotal	17	%

Test II Overall—Total (55 = 20 + 18 + 17): %

For adults, the Tonality Tests are classified into five zones: low, low-mid, mid, mid-high, and high tonality. These are perceptual zones for the spectral pitch of phonemes. All five zones can be used, but for the purpose of simplifying the explanation, only three zones will be used. Each test includes syllables or words that are homogeneous in tonality. For example, /sisi/ has a high-tonality consonant /s/ and high-tonality vowel /i/. The homogeneous selection allows each specific tonality zone to be tested.

If the test items were selected heterogeneously, more than one tonality zone would be targeted at the same time. For example, /mimi/ has a low-tonality consonant /m/ with a high-tonality vowel /i/. The low-tonality zone and the high-tonality zone are tested simultaneously. The heterogeneous test items (e.g., /mimi/) may be easier to perceive than a homogeneous item (e.g., /sisi/). This homogeneous test item of the high-tonality consonant and vowel is the most difficult to perceive.

The Tonality Tests can be nonsense syllables, words, or sentences. For nonsense syllables, the Verbotonal Three-Syllable Test consists of a low (/mumu/), a mid (/lala/), and a high (/sisi/) syllable test item. The zones that are targeted include: below 500 Hz, at 1000 Hz, and above 2000 Hz. If the child does not perceive the high-tonality correctly, he has a high-frequency hearing loss. If he produces an error with the mid- and high-tonality targets (/lala/ and /sisi/, respectively), he has both a mid- and a high-frequency hearing loss, and so on.

For all test items, the child or adult imitates what he or she hears. The client is instructed not to guess. The substitutions and errors made (e.g., /ʃiʃi/ for /sisi/) provide information on which tonality zones are causing problems in perception and production. This has important implications for the treatment strategy, which includes correction through body movements, speech modification, and filter adjustments on the Verbotonal Auditory Training Unit.

The Verbotonal Tonality Words Test has five test words in the low-, mid-, and high-tonality zones. The clinician presents each test word twice, with the client imitating each presentation. The client's imitation is scored as either correct or incorrect, and the specific phonemes produced are transcribed by the clinician. Then, the clinician computes the percent correct for each tonality zone; for example, 100% low, 60% mid, and 20% for high-tonality zones. These results, for example, indicate that the client has a significant perceptual problem in the mid- and high-tonality zones, with a lack of auditory brain transfer to the low-tonality zones. This corresponds to the earlier nonsense syllable results. Both tests usually yield similar results.

The Verbotonal Tonality Sentence Test selects homogeneous tonality words for each sentence. For example, "Pull the Puppy Up" specifically tests the low-tonality zone, because all the words are from the low zone. In contrast, "Tell Tom to Come" is from the mid-tonality zone, and "My Feet Itch" is from the high-tonality zone. All of the sentences have three to four words, and each sentence is scored by the number of correct words. The percent correct within each tonality zone is computed as in the tests described earlier. The sentence test, the word test, and the nonsense test usually show similar results for the zones.

The Tonality Tests are presented without visual cues to measure the client's auditory skills only. All items are presented at the most comfortable loudness (MCL) level to ensure the client's best performance. The tests can be administered to the unaided ear, an ear aided by a hearing aid, and an ear aided by a cochlear implant. The test can be administered in either a quiet or noisy (e.g., +5 dB S/N ratio) environment, and test items can be presented through a speech audiometer in a test booth or at an optimal distance in the therapy room. A skilled Verbotonal clinician establishes reliable test results by speaking each test item at her most comfortable loudness speaking level.

Comparison of Unaided, Aided, and Verbotonal Auditory Training Unit

As mentioned earlier in this chapter, the unaided distance is measured for the child's "better" ear. Using the Fletcher Graph for unaided distance, an estimated optimal listening distance can be predicted. For example, according to the Fletcher Graph, the optimal distance for a 50 dB hearing loss is three feet.

To compare the unaided to the aided condition, the same estimated "optimal distance" is used with and without the hearing aid(s). The percent correct on the Tonality Test is compared for the unaided and aided conditions. The percent correct will be similar if both conditions use the MCL level. The aided condition is then evaluated at a greater distance (e.g., 15 feet). If the hearing aid is programmed properly, the percent correct should be the same (e.g., 80% at 3 feet and 80% at 15 feet). If the scores are similar, the aided condition has increased the child's optimal listening distance to 15 feet while maintaining the same performance outcome (% correct). This is a desired test result.

Optimum Versus Adverse Listening Assessment

The Verbotonal Auditory Training Unit is equipped with reverberation and noise accessories that create adverse listening conditions. These accessories are used after the child demonstrates high performance (e.g., 100%) in the quiet condition. Reverberation time (RT) and noise are used to determine the amount of treatment that is needed to make an adverse listening condition equal to an optimum (quiet) listening condition. The range of reverberation time used is from 0 to 2.2 seconds and the signal-to-noise ratio range is from +30 dB to –15 dB S/N. The assessment for both conditions of reverberation and noise are measured separately to determine the amount of treatment that needs to be focused on each condition. The adverse treatment prepares the child for the poor listening conditions of the mainstream classroom as well as other noisy environments.

Assessment of Adults

For adult assessment, the same tonality procedure described earlier for both cochlear implants (CI) and hearing aids (HA) is used. The analysis of the adult's tonality errors is effective in modifying the CI or HA to improve his performance.

Senior citizens, with or without dementia, usually experience some additional central processing problems. As the adult ages, his brain does not function as efficiently as it did in his younger years; therefore, these older clients usually take longer to process and respond to auditory input. For these adults, the tempo of speech is evaluated separately for slow (two per second), normal (five per second), and fast (eight per second) speech. For older clients, a functional assessment provides useful information for the guiding Verbotonal treatment and for improving the client's performance and satisfaction with his hearing aid(s) and/or cochlear implant.

Verbotonal Auditory Training Unit

The Verbotonal Auditory Training Unit is an advanced digital technology that complements the Verbotonal Approach to treatment. The training unit and the treatment strategy are based on the same principles. The goal for using the unit is to maximize the patient's ability to speak clearly, with normal voice quality, and to be able to understand others in quiet, and eventually noisy and reverberant situations. The training unit allows the Verbotonal clinician to evaluate the client's performance with precise control of the acoustic speech signal.

Bandwidth

The Verbotonal Auditory Training Unit has an extended bandwidth from 2 Hz to 20,000 Hz, covering a 12-octave range. A low-frequency microphone is positioned closely to pick up the clinician's speech patterns of rhythm, intonation, and phonemes. The unit presents the speech input at a pre-established most comfortable loudness (MCL) level through both a high-quality speech vibrator and/or a binaural headset. When the young child responds to the clinician's speech input, the microphone is placed closely to his mouth to maximize his feeling and hearing of his own vocal patterns in comparison to the clinician's vocal patterns. The positioning of the microphone close to the child's mouth also serves as a cue for the young child to imitate the clinician.

The training unit has an extended bandwidth, which is achieved by the speech vibrator's low-frequency range of 2 Hz to 1000 Hz and the binaural headset's large range of 20 Hz to 20,000 Hz. The training unit's total range from 2 Hz to 20,000 Hz covers 12 octaves, which matches the same 12-octave range of the child's brain. This extended bandwidth provides the optimal learning condition for the child's perception of the speech rhythms of both the clinician's voice and the child's own voice.

Matching the extended wide bandwidth to the brain's bandwidth, a Verbotonal strategy, is based on a child developmental model. Most conventional treatment strategies, however, are based on an adult model, in which the bandwidth is narrow (three-octave range), including only the center speech frequencies of a telephone (500–3000 Hz). This adult model promotes the use of hearing aids, emphasizing more amplification of high frequencies, where the hearing loss is the greatest. Unfortunately, in this conventional adult model the clinician has no control over frequency responses or the quality of sound provided by the hearing aids and usually does not have the option of vibrotactile speech input. In contrast, the Verbotonal Approach controls bandwidth, vibrotactile speech input, and the quality of the speech input with the Verbotonal Auditory Training Unit. This strategy uses greater control and is effective in improving listening skills, which is the key to successful oral communication skills.

Loudness

It is very important for young children to have a pleasant experience with speech input, avoiding any pain (recruitment) from excessive use of loudness. Because of the extended wide bandwidth of the Verbotonal Auditory Training Unit, the 12-octave frequency range requires less amplification than a three-octave range. This is because the child is able to "feel" the speech rhythm first, and later hear it. Usually, speech input through the three-octave range of hearing aids is more than 20 dB greater than through the twelve-octave range of the Verbotonal Auditory Training Unit. This additional loudness is often unpleasant, thus creating an unpleasant listening experience for the child.

With the Verbotonal Approach, the most comfortable loudness (MCL) level is adjusted separately for each earphone of the headset and for the speech vibrator on the training unit. Initially, the MCL is established by having the child imitate the clinician's speech rhythm (e.g., /ba ba boo/). By experiencing the speech rhythm vibrotactically through the speech vibrator, the child learns how to listen to the simultaneous auditory input through the headsets. A sound-level meter is used to measure the MCL in the headsets to verify that the MCL is above threshold and that it is not overamplifying the speech signal.

Additionally, using the Verbotonal Auditory Training Unit, the clinician can independently control the loudness level of a bimodal use of low and high frequencies by adjusting the acoustic filter. Both the low and high frequencies can be adjusted in 1-dB steps to ensure the proper balance of both.

Because each young child has a unique MCL level for each ear, normal-hearing children with serious speech problems can be in the same treatment group as a child with a profound hearing loss. The training unit is set for each child individually at his or her unique MCL to maximize access to the clinician's speech patterns and to hear his or her own patterns.

Signal-to-Noise Ratio (S/N)

The Verbotonal Auditory Training Unit provides a quiet (+30 dB) speech signal-to-noise ratio, because the microphone is positioned within three inches of the clinician's or the child's mouth. At a distance of three inches, the speech signal enters the system at 85 dB SPL, which is 30 dB louder than the 65 dB SPL of normal conversational speech, which takes place at an average distance of three feet. This optimal listening condition of a three-inch microphone placement ensures a +30 dB signal-to-noise ratio, because the ambient room noise does not exceed 55 dB SPL (85 dB − 55 dB = 30 dB S/N ratio) in public classrooms or clinics. Therefore, +30 dB S/N ratio is preserved in both the speech vibrator and in the binaural headset, preventing the ambient room noise from interfering with the clinician or child's speech signal. In short, there is no upward spread of masking from low-frequency room noise to high-frequency speech sounds.

Some treatment strategies advocate "leaning over" or sitting beside the child's hearing-aid microphone, but this is not practical and does not represent a natural listening situation. The Verbotonal strategy is to sit in front of the child while using the Verbotonal Auditory Training Unit to aid in the transmission of the speech signal. In this position, the clinician covers her face while speaking to reduce visual cues. This condition allows the child to maximize his listening skills. Together, the clinician's speech input and the Verbotonal Auditory Training Unit provide the optimal listening condition for learning.

Consistent Amplification

The consistent daily use of a wide bandwidth in a +30 dB S/N ratio provides the optimum learning condition for the young child to perceive and internalize speech rhythms. This is why the Verbotonal Auditory Training Unit is so important; it is an effective tool in establishing the body-ear link necessary for the child's speech processing.

The training unit is always available for the treatment session, and it is not dependent on the parent or child for proper functioning, as is a hearing aid, which requires frequent battery changes. This consistent use of quality amplification and vibrotactile speech input provided by the training unit is critical during the limited time windows of normal development of listening skills and speech skills.

Cochlear Implant Strategy

An effective "precochlear implant" strategy can be implemented by stimulating the child's brain with normal speech rhythm. The Verbotonal Auditory Training Unit, with vibrotactile speech input and binaural headset stimulation, provides an optimal learning and treatment condition. In this optimal condition, the clinician can evaluate the child's potential for continuing hearing-aid use at home or opting for a cochlear implant.

If a parent chooses a cochlear implant for his or her child, the brain's processing of speech rhythms will provide the foundation for his successful use of the cochlear implant. After the cochlear implant has been implanted, the training unit is used to provide vibrotactile speech input. This way the child can feel speech through the training unit and hear speech through his cochlear implant. In addition, a monaural headset can be placed on the child's contralateral ear to help develop binaural processing of speech. With the Verbotonal Auditory Training Unit, the child's success with his cochlear implant is enhanced, which increases the possibility for him to be successfully mainstreamed.

Vibrotactile to Air Conduction

As previously mentioned, an infant initially receives vibrotactile speech input by being placed on a vibrating board on the floor or in his crib. The board has three vibrators attached to the underside of it. When the clinician, parent, or infant vocalizes, the infant feels the speech rhythms through his entire body; this is known as body perception. In this condition, a preword dialogue is established; the clinician or parent imitates the infant's babbling, and the infant attempts to imitate the clinician's or parent's vocal patterns. This preword dialogue is the basis for the development of higher level language and more complex speech dialogue.

As treatment progresses, a separate speech vibrator is attached with a Velcro band to the infant's leg or arm, similar to a wristwatch. When the infant sits upright and begins to crawl, one or two speech vibrators are attached, and the vibration board is no longer needed. When the young child can regularly wear the binaural headset, he begins to hear through the headset what was previously "felt" through the vibrators. This is the beginning of establishing auditory dominance. This usually occurs when the young child can imitate and remember rhythm and intonation patterns of three to six syllables, with normal voice quality. The earphones provide more speech information than the vibrators, so when his speech rhythm patterns are stable, the speech vibrators can be phased out.

With consistent vibrotactile speech input, the clinician usually observes a significant improvement in the infant's voice quality and speech rhythm processing. Over the past 40 years of implementing the Verbotonal Approach, no cases of tactual or headset defensiveness have been reported. The clinician is skilled in creating a situation in which wearing the speech vibrator and the binaural headset is a pleasant experience for the child. Often receiving treatment in small groups, the children do what the other children are doing. This peer bonding helps the children accept these new and unfamiliar treatment conditions.

Spectral Speech Changes

After a series of successive treatment sessions, children will respond favorably to spectral changes (acoustic filters) in the Verbotonal Auditory Training Unit. For example, a 600 Hz low-pass filter emphasizes the rhythm and intonation pattern essential for learning and remembering the speech rhythm. This filter also prepares a restructuring of hearing through an auditory brain transfer through the low frequencies.

For bimodal spectral changes, a low-pass filter and a high-pass filter are combined simultaneously to improve the processing and verbalizing of speech. The low-pass filter is the most important component because it emphasizes the rhythm and intonation patterns of speech, which enhances the child's perception of high-frequency speech energy.

Controlling Speech Spectrum with Pivotal Frequencies and Slopes

Each filter in the Verbotonal Auditory Training Unit has a slope and a center frequency. For example, the low-pass filter has discrete center frequencies from 90 Hz to 4000 Hz, with each center frequency having slopes of 0, 6, 12, or 18 dB/octave toward lows, and slopes of 20 or 60 dB/octave toward highs. With a center frequency of 1000 Hz, a 6-dB slope drops 6 dB at 500 Hz, 6 dB at 250 Hz, 6 dB at 125 Hz, and so forth. In other words, from 1000 to 125 Hz, the signal drops a total of 18 dB. This low-frequency slope is critical in the child's development. As a child's listening skills progress, he or she needs less low-frequency energy. The Verbotonal Auditory Training Unit offers a broader range of possibilities needed by clients with hearing loss. The training unit offers the advantage to use acoustic filters to control the acoustics of the speech signal input (see Figures 3–2 and 3–3).

With the Verbotonal Approach, all infants begin with a broad bandwidth that extends from 2 Hz to 20,000 Hz to fully stimulate the young brain's wide bandwidth. In a normal mother-infant interaction, the mother's wide speech spectrum is presented through the Verbotonal Auditory Training Unit. After the infant internalizes normal rhythm and intonation patterns, fewer low speech frequencies are needed so a downward slope of 6 dB or 12 dB/octave is used. The 20 dB or 60 dB/octave slopes toward the highs are used to make a large separation (60 dB/octave) or a small separation (20 dB/octave) between the low speech frequencies and high speech frequencies.

The slopes and the center frequency are set first, because the low frequencies provides rhythm and intonation patterns. The low-pass section has 12 center frequencies, whereas the high-pass section has only four center frequencies. The additional center frequencies are needed so the clinician can select the optimal amount of lows for each child and make the appropriate modifications as the child's listening skills progress.

The high-pass filter section has four center frequencies (2, 3, 4, and 6 kHz), with 20 dB or 60 dB/octave slopes toward lows, and 0 dB or

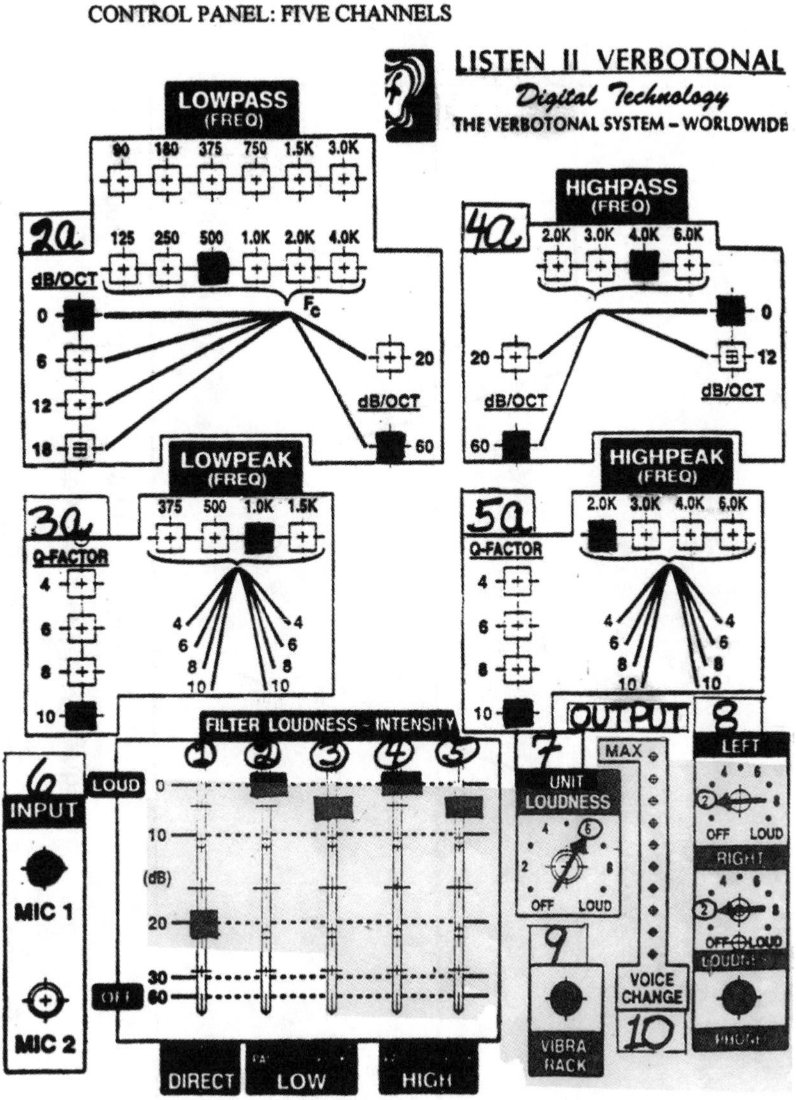

CONTROL PANEL: FIVE CHANNELS

Figure 3–2. Five-Channel Control Unit Panel

12 dB/octave slopes toward highs. As mentioned earlier, the 60 dB/octave create a large separation, and the 20 dB/octave create a small separation between high and low frequencies.

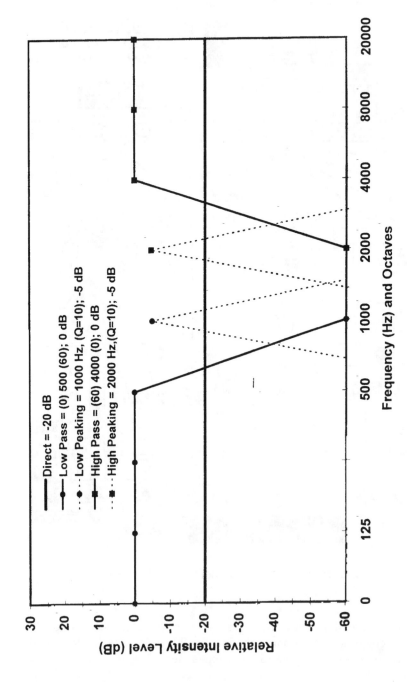

Figure 3–3. Frequency responses of the Five Channels

The Verbotonal Auditory Training Unit, used in group treatment session, has a broad bandwidth and a low-pass filter. The unit used most often in individual treatment has five channels: broadband, low-pass, high-pass, low-peaking, and high-peaking filters. All five channels can be activated at different loudness levels, with the loudest band, usually the low-pass, set at the child's most comfortable loudness (MCL) level. The other bands are equal to or less than the MCL level; the less-loudness bands are noted as –5, –10, –20 dB, and so forth. A notation system is used to identify the exact listening condition (optimum frequency response) that was used.

Spectral Changes: The Notation System

The notation system for the Verbotonal Auditory Training Unit includes the center frequency (Hz), the slopes (dB/octaves), and the loudness (dB) used. A low-pass plus high-pass filter bimodal condition would be: LP: (0) 1000 (60) = 0 dB, HP: (60) 4000 (0) = –5dB. If the other three bands were used, they would be: BB (broadband) = –20 dB, LB (low-band) = –5 dB, and HB (high-band) –5 dB. By appropriately changing the loudness levels (dB) of the five channels, the child's brain learns to perceive lows more than highs or at least to perceive them equally. The loudness level of the broadband can range from the highest, most dominant loudness level (MCL = 0 dB) to the least loudness level (–60 dB). The least loudness of –60 dB maximizes the brain's perception of the optimum frequency response set with the filters. The dominant broadband (BB) level to the least loudness level varies the "background" of the BB in developing the child's listening skills.

Optimal Frequency Response

The optimal frequency response (OFR) always begins with the broadband (BB). The first filter condition is the low-pass filter, because it includes the rhythm and intonation of the clinician's and the child's vocal patterns. The progressive steps are:

Step 1 = BB   (All Frequency Listening)

Step 2 = LP (0 dB slope)   (Low Transfer)

Step 3 = LP (6 dB or 12 dB) + HP   (Bimodal)

   (3a) For example, 750 LP plus 4K high-pass

   (3b) For example, 1000 LP plus 2000 HP

Step 4 = BB added to Step 2 or Step 3

(4a) = at –6 dB for digital hearing aid or cochlear implant users

(4b) = MCL for normal hearing cases who have an auditory process-
       ing disorder (APD)

The above four OFR steps can take 1 to 12 weeks with easy cases, or 1 to 6 years for difficult cases. The listening progression is similar regardless of the severity of the case; it is the rate of progression that varies.

New Digital Technology Models

The Verbotonal Auditory Training Units (VATU) come in a variety of models, but all the models are based on the same Verbotonal treatment strategy. Model 1 has two channels (BB + LP), whereas Model 2 has five channels (BB + LP + HP + LB + HB). Model 1 is used as the rhythm and intonation levels for young children in groups (6-10 children) or in individual treatment. Model 2 can be used as Model 1, or it can be used at the phoneme level in group or individual sessions. The difference between the two models is that Model 2 is more effective at the phoneme and word level. Model 3 is slightly different; its low-fre-quency and high-frequency narrow bands are one-octave wide versus peaking filters. This model has some advantages for adjusting the opti-mal octaves. Model 4 is a unique 3-channel combination of both spec-tral (filter) and temporal (delays) information. The temporal delays between the low-pass and high-pass filters vary between 0 msec and 1 second. These delays are especially effective with severe speech dis-orders (i.e., aphasia and stuttering) and for teaching foreign language and pronunciation. All four models have the current digital technology that is compatible with all digital hearing aids and cochlear implants.

Some VATU models are portable, with a carrying case, and are user-friendly. All VATUs have a lifetime of 40 years and excellent main-tenance records.

Accessories

As with the Verbotonal Auditory Training Unit (VATU), the accessories are of high quality. The microphones are modern electrocondenser microphones with an adjustable "gooseneck." The clinician wears an attractive breastplate that positions the microphone close to his or her mouth. As mentioned earlier, this close position (within 3 inches) creates a quiet listening condition (+30 dB S/N) for the child. The clinician can easily remove the microphone and hold it near the child to ensure the same quiet listening condition for when the child is listening to his own vocalizations. For signal output, the VATU includes a speech vibrator and a binaural headset for each child. With an infant, the clinician uses a vibrating board, and at later stages attaches the vibrator to the child's wrist.

The binaural headsets are circumaural and are positioned around the client's ears. This position creates a 30 dB reduction in the room noise (i.e., a 55-dB room noise will be attenuated to a comparable 25-dB level). The circumaural design also serves as a resonator for the low-frequency speech energy of the clinician's voice. The low-frequency emphasis of the electrocondenser microphone, the circumaural headset, and the speech vibrator all help to provide an extended low-frequency response to match the wide bandwidth of the child's brain.

The clinician uses a VATU with one or two five-station racks, with each station having three loudness adjustments. Adjustments can be made to the left ear, right ear, and the vibrator, independently. One rack provides simultaneous stimulation to five children, whereas two racks provide it for ten children.

The clinician uses a sound level meter (SLM) to verify and calibrate the loudness (dB) level used in each earphone. For example, a SLM speech measure of 80 dB SPL is converted to a 60 dB HL (−20 dB) to determine if the 60 dB HL is compatible to the child's speech reception threshold (SRT) and if it is a most comfortable loudness level (MCL) in that ear.

The SLM provides an accurate verification of the clinician's and the child's vocal pattern and a verification of MCL. The SLM ensures the appropriate loudness level and minimizes the chances of overamplification. This results in a pleasant listening experience for the child.

The Verbotonal Auditory Training Units are hardwired systems with special cords connecting the microphone, the speech vibrators, and the binaural headsets to the Unit. The hardwires conveniently restrict the group space to a radius of 15 feet. The restricted space keeps a group of six to ten children under control and helps the group learn to work as a team. The clinician's voice is set louder than the other children in the group, so that her voice is the "model voice" and so that she can lead the activities. In some cases, the treatment condition can be less restrictive when it is possible to use a wireless microphone.

Cochlear Implants and Hearing Aids—Treatment

With the development of advanced digital technology, the prognosis is excellent for improving the processing and verbalizing of speech for all types of communication problems. This new digital technology has resulted in the development of cochlear implants, advances in hearing aids, and modernizing the Verbotonal Auditory Training Units (VATU). To achieve and fulfill an excellent prognosis for a child with hearing loss, it is important to stimulate the child's brain with the optimal learning conditions, using the appropriate new technology.

New Technology—Cochlear Implants

1. **Digitizing Speech**—With new digital technology, it is possible to instantaneously transfer normal conversational speech into a digital code for computer processing. The computer has unlimited possibilities for modifying the code and presenting it to the child's brain. The biggest challenge is selecting the code that is optimal for each learning stage of the child's brain processing of auditory input.

2. **Miniaturizing the Cochlear Implant**—The cochlear implant technology has evolved from a "body-worn" speech processor to a "behind-the-ear" speech processor. This developmental evolution will follow with an "in-the-ear" processor and later a completely implantable "under the skin" processor. All of these developmental stages are possible because of the miniaturization of digital electronics. This is cosmetically attractive to the user, as it is less noticeable as being different from people with normal hearing.

3. **Basic Components**—The microphone on the speech processor picks up the speech signal of the speaker as well as the environmental noise. The speech signal is digitized by the speech processor, transmitted through an electromagnet (both sides of the skin of the mastoid) and activated through an electrode that has been surgically placed in the left or right cochlea. The surgeon follows a standard surgical procedure of inserting the electrode into the cochlea and positioning it near the modiolus. The modiolus is the central core of the cochlea that contains the spiral ganglia, a collection of cell bodies of afferent (input) auditory nerve fibers that are found after the hair cells of the cochlea and before the auditory nerve.

Because there is hair cell damage in a sensorineural hearing loss, the close positioning of the implanted electrodes is important for direct electrical stimulation of these spiral ganglia cell bodies. The idea is to bypass the damaged hair cells and directly stimulate the spiral ganglia (auditory nerve).

The length of the electrode array and the insertion distance of the electrode are important for creating a broad bandwidth for the tonotopic organization of the frequencies. One cochlear implant (CI) company advertises an extra long electrode (31 mm) with full insertion to the apex of the cochlea to stimulate the low frequencies of rhythm and intonation of speech.

The speech processor can be programmed (mapped) for up to 22 channels, covering a frequency range of 300 Hz to 5000 Hz. However, if the speech processor is to stimulate the wide response of the cochlea, 20 Hz to 20,000 Hz, the processor and the electrodes need to cover that entire range (20 Hz to 20,000 Hz) of the cochlea. Because the tonotopic organization from the cochlea to the brain connects at all neural levels, the tonotopic stimulation through the cochlea is important for "high-fidelity" hearing. This organization is achieved by the major components of the cochlear implant: the microphone, the speech processor, the electromagnetic couplers, and the implanted electrode array.

4. **Mapping: Programming the Speech Processor**—After the patient has recovered from the surgical implant, an audiologist "turns on" the CI by adjusting the detection thresholds and most comfortable loudness levels in each channel of the processor. A computer is linked to the CI to make these adjustments. In young infants and toddlers, the thresholds are set based on behavioral responses (e.g., eye blinking) of the infant. This is a very difficult process and sometimes unpleasant for the young child. For an adult CI user, the mapping process is much easier because the adult can consciously respond to each sound and describe its characteristics.

New Technology—Hearing Aid(s)

Conventional hearing aids have evolved from a body-worn model to an in-the-canal model over the past 50 years. As with cochlear implants, the hearing aids have the new programmable digital technology and are miniaturized to fit in the ear canal. The computer, interfaced with the digital hearing aid, is used to adjust the independent channels of the hearing aid for each client. Digital hearing aids and cochlear implants are very similar in how new technology has affected the "fitting" or "programming" strategies. With the new technologic advances, more options are available for aligning the output with the tonotopic organization from the cochlea to the brain.

Residual Hearing: Can It Be Functional?

Over the past two hundred years, numerous authors have emphasized the importance of residual hearing. Most professionals agree on its importance; however, how to specifically identify and develop residual hearing is not clear.

Technically, the residual hearing is the hearing sensitivity that remains after a hearing loss that is caused by sensorineural cochlear damage. The hearing sensitivity is measured by pure-tone detection thresholds between 125 Hz and 8000 Hz. Typically, most clients have high-frequency hearing loss in the 2000 Hz to 8000 Hz region and demonstrate better hearing in the low-frequency range of 125 Hz to 1000 Hz. The low frequencies may have 20 dB HL to 80 dB HL more sensitivity than the high frequencies. Anatomically, the upper apical part of the cochlea shows more sensitivity in the low frequencies, whereas the lower basal part shows more sensitivity to the high frequencies. This information is important to understanding the tonotopic organization of the frequencies within the cochlea.

The Verbotonal Strategy has been successful because it has focused on maximizing the more sensitive low-frequency zones and making them functional. To become functional, the low frequency residual hearing is stimulated with the Verbotonal Auditory Training Units to develop the child's natural perceptual transfer. This treatment strategy of developing the most sensitive frequency zones is also used for hearing aid placement, which begins with the Verbotonal broad bandwidth hearing aid(s). The frequency response of the hearing aid(s) always includes the low frequencies (125 to 1000 Hz) to maximize the brain's perception of the rhythm and intonation of speech. As was discussed earlier in the text, the rhythm and intonation of speech provide the foundation for perceiving the 43 American phonemes.

In contrast, most conventional hearing aid placement strategies follow the "mirroring" of the hearing loss. This mirroring implies the largest amplification (gain in dB) in the high-frequency region with the greatest hearing loss, and the smallest amplification in the low-frequency region. In fact, the "mirroring" does not include the low frequencies because of the "fear" of a potential "upward spread of masking." This fear is that environmental noise may interfere (mask) with the high-frequency consonants that are "weaker." This conventional assumption asserts that vowels are in the lows and consonants are in the highs. This is in contrast to the Verbotonal Strategy of the tonalities where vowels and consonants cover the entire range from lows to highs (i.e., /i/ is a high tonality vowel and /b/ is a low tonality consonant), and the Verbotonal Auditory Training Unit treatment in the quiet condition (+30 dB S/N) avoids any upward spread of masking from environmental noise.

As a result, conventional hearing aid placement, without treatment, amplifies the high frequencies with the idea of restoring "normal hearing." The goal is an aided pure-tone threshold of 25 dB HL or less through the hearing aid in a sound field. However, to reach a 95 dB HL unaided threshold at 4000 Hz, it takes 70 dB of amplification to achieve a 25 dB HL threshold ($95 - 70 = 25$). The problem with this conventional policy is that, with unaided thresholds of 70 dB HL or greater, there is a "perceptual distortion" in the "dead zones" for the high amplification levels, because of the hair cell damage in the cochlea. The aided thresholds of 25 dB HL is seldom achieved in this example.

Because normal-hearing native speakers can communicate with the narrow bandwidth of the telephone, researchers have assumed that hearing-impaired children can communicate in a similar narrow bandwidth. The narrow bandwidth of the telephone, the radio, and the televison is cheaper to market than a wide high-fidelity bandwidth. Most professionals use the telephone strategy for hearing-impaired clients by amplifying a narrow bandwidth in the area of greatest hearing loss. These are called high-frequency hearing aids and do not include the suprasegmental patterns of speech. The Verbotonal Strategy is different in that it emphasizes the area of the residual hearing. The complex question is what frequency region of the residual hearing should be emphasized, should it be made functional, and what role does the client's brain play in the speech processing? The Verbotonal Strategy addresses these questions.

In comparison, the cochlear implant strategy is different than working with hearing aids because the electrical stimulation in the cochlea is assumed to bypass the damaged hair cell and to stimulate the spiral ganglia cells directly. However, the CI strategy needs to take advantage of the more sensitive low-frequency residual hearing, especially when the treatment has developed the brain perception of speech rhythm through the lows.

Generally, the CI aided thresholds are relatively flat at 30 dB HL from 500 to 4000 Hz. These flat thresholds are better than most hearing-aid-aided thresholds, but are still not "normal thresholds" of 0 dB HL. Also, the monaural CI is a unilateral implant.

Comparison of Cochlear Implants and Hearing Aids

For profound hearing losses, the most recent research has demonstrated a considerable advantage (+30%) of CIs over hearing aids for both children and adults. This advantage is understandable because hearing aids have not been successful with profound hearing loss. For example, most residential schools for the deaf have children who do not have understandable speech and cannot use their hearing for communication or as the main modality for communicating and learning. As a result, most of these children are forced to use a manual form of communication. For these children, the amplification of the hearing aid(s) is not sufficient by itself. The type of treatment for these children should be evaluated to determine if it improves performance outcome with the hearing aid(s).

In comparison to hearing aids, some professionals view CIs as "restoring normal hearing." If so, it is more reasonable to compare CIs outcome performance to the performance of normal-hearing children and adults of similar ages. This "benchmark" of normal hearing may be a better indication of the child's success. However, CIs have had a significant positive impact on improving the listening skills of the hearing-impaired children and adults, improving their quality of life and creating interest in the type and auditory strategy of the treatment. The challenge is what auditory treatment strategy produces the best performance outcome?

Verbotonal Auditory Training Units (VATU)

As mentioned earlier, the Verbotonal Auditory Training Unit (VATU) with the newest digital technology is used to create the optimal frequency response. This begins with the broad bandwidth to stimulate the child's brain and moves to a bimodal optimal frequency response (OFR). Then, a smooth and successful transition is made from the VATU to the cochlear implant or hearing aid, with the child maintaining a similar performance level. This is possible because all the units have digital technology for fine tuning for the frequency response. The next section describes this unique treatment strategy.

Transition from VATU to the Cochlear Implant or Hearing Aid

From Vibrotactile Input to Air-Conduction

The Verbotonal prehearing aid and precochlear implant treatment strategies both use the vibrotactile speech input from the VATU to allow the infant to "feel" the natural speech rhythm of the trainer, the mother, and his or her voice. At first, these rhythms are felt through the infant's body by laying or sitting the infant on a vibrating speech board. Once the infant-toddler can consistently imitate the speech rhythms, there is a transition from vibrotactile input to air-conduction input through the binaural headphones (i.e., the infant "hears" what he or she felt"). Hearing through the headphones prepares the infant for hearing through the cochlear implant or hearing aid(s) because the infant can respond to setting either device. This makes the transition a pleasant experience for the child.

The vibrotactile stimulation for the infant needs to be introduced carefully, so the infant realizes the connection between what he or she feels and the clinician's voice. Then, the infant learns that his or her voice also creates a pleasant feeling of speech rhythm and that he or she can control others with voice. The child establishes a dialogue with the clinician and his or her mother. This link is important for the transition from vibrotactile speech input to the air-conduction speech signal.

Spectral and Temporal Speech Change with VATU

After the speech rhythm foundation and the hearing are established, the VATU is used to create spectral (bimodal) and temporal (time delay) changes to facilitate the child's processing and verbalizing of the phonemes, syllables, and words. This develops the cochlea to brain tonotopic organization.

The optimal frequency response (OFR) on the VATU is used for the programming of the cochlear implant's speech processor. The program in the processor can be used for treatment because its performance is similar to the VATU. Essentially, the VATU prepares the child's brain for either the CI or the hearing aid(s) to maximize the child's processing through that device.

Treatment with Cochlear Implants and Hearing Aids

For the hearing aid users, the VATU binaural headsets and speech vibrator are used in treatment and the hearing aids are used after/outside of treatment. This treatment provides a "positive" learning transfer to the hearing aids. For example, a +20% improvement in VATU treatment, results in a 15 to 20% improvement in the hearing aid(s).

For the cochlear implant users, the CI is always used in the treatment sessions. However, the vibrotactile input from the VATU is used to develop the child's voice, rhythm, intonation patterns, and phoneme processing. The vibrotactile speech input is used as long as it provides the optimal learning condition and the child improves.

Because the CI is a monaural speech input, coming from only one earphone, the VATU headsets is used on the child's contralateral ear. The development of the unimplanted ear should help the child's binaural listening and may prepare the ear for a hearing aid or a second CI. The final goal is to make the child a binaural listener and have a binaural advantage in adverse listening conditions.

The new technology of the VATU is compatible with the new technology of both CI and HA, and it provides a strategy to maximize the child's performance and outcome. Every parent expects his or her child to both speak clearly and understand what others have said. This new technology and treatment strategy make this possible for both children and adults.

Technology for Reverberation and Noise

The Verbotonal Strategy stressed the importance of providing the optimal learning condition to stimulate the child's brain and complete the normal learning process. For example, a quiet condition (+30 dB HL S/N) is optimal for learning, but what happens when the child or adult is confronted with adverse listening conditions? The Verbotonal treatment strategy for the adverse conditions is discussed next.

Reverberation

Research has documented the adverse effects of both noise and reverberation on listening and speech communication. In a one-to-one speech dialogue at a close distance of 3 feet, an adverse listening condition (i.e., a loud TV program) has a minimal impact, but at greater distances of 6 to 20 feet, it degrades the client's speech understanding by 40 to 60%. These greater distances occur in most public school classrooms and in social and recreational situations. As reverberation is not well understood by most practitioners, it will be discussed first.

In normal speech dialogue, the talker's speech comes to the listener(s) through both a direct sound and a reflected sound. The direct sound decreases in loudness (dB) by 6 dB every time the distance is doubled in free space. For example, at a normal dialogue distance of 3 feet, the talker's speech level is 65 dB SPL; however, at 6 feet, it is 59 dB; at 12 feet, it is 53 dB; at 24 feet, it is 49 dB, and so on. At three feet, the talker's loudness is comfortable (MCL) to the listener. However, at 24 feet the talker's loudness may be too soft for the listener to understand what the talker said. Even though it is direct sound, the talker-to-listener distance is a factor in both quiet and in adverse listening conditions.

In an enclosed room, there is reverberation of the talker's voice as it is reflected off the walls, ceiling, and floor. The reverberation is defined as the persistence of the sound in an enclosed room as a result of multiple speech reflections. It can be measured by the size (volume) of the room and the absorption of the room surfaces. Typically, a larger room with more reflection has a greater reverberation time (RT) than a smaller room. The RT is the time in seconds for a sound to decrease 60 dB after the sound source has stopped. For example, for a RT of 0.2 seconds, it takes 0.2 seconds for the talker's voice of 65 dB SPL to decrease to 5 dB SPL. Typically, the RT ranges from no reverberation to a long reverberation of 2.2 seconds.

An RT of 2.2 seconds would occur in a large cathedral, performance hall, or basketball gym with hard surfaces (walls, ceiling, floors). In adverse listening conditions, it would be difficult to understand the talker(s). Whereas, a small comfortable room in a home with soft surfaces and rugs, wooden furniture, and so forth may have a 0.2 RT. In this small room, it would be easy to understand the talker(s).

To estimate the listener's difficulty of different size rooms, the "critical distance" (CD) is used for this estimate. The CD is the distance at which the direct and the reflected sound have the same loudness (dB). For example, at a normal dialogue distance of three feet, the direct sound from the talker to the listener is louder (65 dB SPL) than the reflected sound (59 dB SPL). However, at 6 feet, the direct sound (59 dB) and the reflected sound (59 dB) are equal in loudness; at 12 feet the direct sound is softer (53 dB) than the reflected sound (59 dB). In this example, the critical distance is at 6 feet where the loudness is equal. The listener would be advised to sit at a distance less than 6 feet. The listener's understanding would be better at 3 feet than at 6 feet because the direct sound is 6 dB louder than the reflected sound.

If the CD is applied to a public school classroom, all children should sit less than 6 feet from the teacher, if possible. However, if the child has a hearing loss or a speech (auditory) processing disorder (APD), he or she should sit even closer.

Some public school classrooms have been modified to minimize the adverse effects of reverberation. These modifications usually include soft rugs and curtains, special soft textured walls and ceilings, and so forth. This reduces the reverberation time and increases the critical distance. Another modification is for the teacher to wear a wireless microphone that is connected to an amplifier/loudspeaker system. This system increases the loudness of the direct sound, and minimizes the affect of the reflective sounds. However, these modifications are expensive and may not be available in all classrooms.

Noise

Noise is defined as any undesired sound, or unwanted disturbance, that interferes with speech communication between a talker (teacher) and a listener (child). The noise can be aperiodic or periodic. Most environmental noise is aperiodic, such as a window air conditioner. The air conditioner is important for cooling, but the noise is not meaningful and it disturbs communication in the classroom. On the other hand, the voiceless fricative consonants of speech (i.e., /f,s/) are aperiodic, but they are meaningful phonemes that are needed to understand the speech of the teacher. So, being aperiodic does not define a signal as noise or important speech energy.

In a "cocktail party" situation, many people are all speaking at the same time. There may be 10 to 20 independent dialogues going on at the same time in the same room. For a listener, these competing dialogues interfere with his listening to one talker. In order to focus on one talker, the listener needs to ignore the other dialogues. To simulate a "cocktail party" effect, ten talkers were recorded while speaking at the same time. This is referred to as "babble noise" because it sounds like a background of babble. A good normal hearing listener can "tune in" to one of the talkers, or "tune out" all of the talkers and listen only to the person in dialogue with him. The babble noise does not affect his or her listening skills.

However, children with attention deficit disorder (ADD) and/or a hearing impairment usually have difficulty listening in noise, because they are distracted by the many talkers and they cannot focus on one voice. The ability to tune in or tune out the unwanted noise is a skill that has to be learned, can be improved, and is necessary for effective normal communication in adverse listening situations. In short, should we change every room in the child's environment, or should we improve his or her listening skills for adverse listening conditions?

Optimal to Adverse Listening Conditions

The Verbotonal Auditory Training Units (VATU) have accessories to control both the reverberation and noise under the binaural headsets and through the speech vibrator. This is a unique treatment technology to control the optimumal to adverse listening conditions. The technology can simulate a small quiet room or a large reverberant area with or without noise.

One accessory is a reverberation unit (RU) that is attached to the microphone input to the VATU. The RU can be adjusted from 0 to 2.2 reverberation time (RT). At RT = 0 seconds, there is no reverberation, whereas at RT = 2.2 seconds, it has the maximum reverberation of a large gymnasium.

The treatment begins by selecting the optimal learning condition which is usually RT = 0 seconds. Then, during a 30-minute treatment session, the RT is gradually increased from the optimum to an adverse listening condition (i.e., RT = 0.6 seconds).

The clinician uses the error analysis procedure described earlier to analyze the child's responses. In her next presentation to the child, she includes her voice modification, body movement(s), and spectral and/or temporal changes in the VATU. Her modifications will help the child improve, and make the adverse listening condition (RT = 0.6 seconds) seem like the optimal learning condition (RT = 0 seconds). When this happens in this learning process, the child's performance (100% correct) in both the adverse and the optimal learning condition is equal. Now, the child's optimal range has increased from 0.0 to 0.6 seconds. With additional treatment, the child's optimal range may increase to 2.2 seconds. This means that the child's listening performance is the same or similar at a variety of reverberation times, or, said another way, in small or large rooms.

The VATU also has an accessory for noise input from a compact disk player. The treatment sessions begin with the aperiodic white noise because it is an easier listening condition. The clinician begins with the optimum learning condition of quiet of +30 dB S/N as she talks to the child. As she increases the white noise in 5-dB steps, the optimum changes to the adverse listening condition. As a result, the child's listening performance gets poorer (i.e., 100% goes to 60%). As with the reverberation treatment, the clinician uses voice modification, body movements, and spectral and temporal changes in the VATU. The clinician's modifications improve the child's performance in the adverse listening condition to 100% correct. As before, the adverse becomes an optimum condition. After the child's optimum is "stretched" from +30 dB to +5 dB S/N, the clinician changes the compact disk player to the babble noise, which is the ten talkers, speaking at the same time. This babble noise is used in the training sessions from +30 dB to +5 dB S/N.

After "stretching" the optimum in both reverberation and noise, the clinician uses both reverberation and noise at the same time, in the graduated steps described above. When a child's performance is 100% correct with RT = 2.2 seconds and a +5 dB S/N, the child or the adult should be successful with all listening conditions at school, recreation, social, and home. This represents the "true" complete mainstreaming of the child's listening skills.

In short, the clinicians use the VATU accessories of reverberation and noise to expand the child's optimal learning condition to everyday adverse listening conditions. This helps make the child a confident and successful listener, who is not in need of a specially treated room.

References

Asp, C. W. (1999) *Tonality Syllable, Word and Sentence Tests.* Unpublished tests, Verbotonal Speech Science Research Laboratory, University of Tennessee, Knoxville, TN.

Asp, C. W., & Plyler, P. (1999). The use of PB and tonality words to optimize hearing aid setting. *Audiology Today, 10,* 27–29.

Bredberg, G. (1968). Cellular pattern and nerve supply of the human organ of corti. *Acta Otolaryngolica, 236.*

Guberina, P. (1972). *The correlation between sensitivity of the vestibular system, and hearing and speech in Verbotonal rehabilitation* (Appendix 6, pp. 256–260). Washington, DC: Office of Vocational Rehabilitation, Department of Health, Education, and Welfare.

Kim, Y., & Asp, C. W. (2002). Low frequency perception of rhythm and intonation speech patterns by normal hearing adults. *Korean Journal of Speech Sciences, 9*(1), 9–16.

Koike, K., & Asp, C. W. (1982). Tennessee test of rhythm and intonation patterns. *Journal of Speech and Hearing Disorders, 46,* 81–87.

Miner, R., & Danhauer, J. (1977). Relationship between formant frequencies and optimal octaves in vowel perception. *American Audiology Society, 2*(5), 163–168.

CHAPTER

4

Speech Strategy: Foundation with Rhythm and Intonation Patterns

One goal of the Verbotonal Approach is to develop good voice quality and intelligible conversational speech that is based on rhythm and intonation patterns. These patterns are the foundation for the perception and production of natural spoken language and well-developed listening skills.

During the babbling and jargon stages of development, an infant with normal hearing begins to express and communicate his or her needs and emotions. The mother is able to understand her infant because the infant's vocalizations are rich in meaning. In turn, the infant is able to understand his mother's speech patterns, which carry an exaggerated intonation, a reduced tempo, and high-pitched rhythm patterns. A meaningful situational dialogue is established between the mother and her infant. The mother's love is conveyed through her speech patterns, facial expressions, and close body contact, creating a situation of emotional security and encouragement to use speech to communicate.

The Verbotonal Approach encourages the child to listen and imitate the preword rhythm and intonation patterns of the clinician. For example, the clinician produces the speech model /ma ma ma (pause) ma/. The child then imitates the clinician's model (Kim & Asp, 2002;

Koike & Asp, 1982). The child's pattern is correct if he or she accurately reproduces the unique rhythm and intonation pattern of the clinician's model. To expand the child's mean length of utterance, the clinician gradually increases the number of syllables in his speech model to stretch the child's auditory memory span.

As part of the treatment plan, the clinician uses a stimulus-response paradigm with indirect correction to target the child's perceptual errors. After analyzing his error(s), the clinician uses the seven speech parameters to create an appropriate speech modification to improve the child's auditory perception and vocal response. For example, if the child substituted /b/ for the target phoneme /m/, his error analysis indicates that the child's /b/ error has more tension and a shorter duration than the target /m/. The greater tension within the child's body forces him to produce and perceive a more tense /b/. To correct the child's error, the clinician uses a less tense body movement and a longer duration while producing the target /m/, along with providing vibrotactile speech input. The body movement and vibrotactile input help the child feel the longer duration and decreased tension of /m/; this helps facilitate the perception and production of the less tense /m/. If the child continues to make the /b/ error, the clinician changes his speech model to the syllable /am/. With the /m/ in the final position, the tension is reduced even more, making it more likely to be perceived correctly. Once correct perception and production are achieved, the clinician reintroduces the original model of /ma/ with the least amount of tension possible. This type of perceptual training, which targets the correction of the specific speech error, helps the child perceive, produce, and remember the correct response. Once this correct response is firmly established in treatment, the child should generalize the correct production to everyday situations.

Another treatment tool is to use situational dialogue to highlight the pragmatics of spoken language. Each situational dialogue involves a story of two or more characters. The situation should be interesting, fun, and meaningful to the child. At first, the child observes the clinician acting out the dialogue. Later, he or she will attempt the speech dialogue by role-playing one or more characters in the story. For example, the characters mommy, daddy, and baby have the dialogue: "Hi, Baby. Where's your Daddy? Here's Daddy. Let's go for a walk. Walk-walk-walk. Bye, Daddy. Come home soon." This type of situational dialogue indirectly teaches social interaction. This early development of pragmatics increases the child's conversational and social skills that are critical for successful mainstreaming.

Rhythm and Intonation Speech Patterns

The term "suprasegmentals" was originally used with written language, whereby the reader supraimposes his or her unique rhythm and intonation speech patterns while orally reading the written words, sentences, and paragraphs, bringing "life" to the words. The "supra" refers to placing the rhythm and intonation "on top of" the written words.

In contrast, the term "segmental" is applied to the 26 alphabet letters that are used to spell out each word, sentence, paragraph, and so forth. These segmental are restricted to each written letter; whereas, the spoken suprasegmentals apply to more than one spoken "segment." For example, the word "ought" can be spoken with an upward intonation pattern that gradually rises across the five alphabet letters. In short, suprasegmental speech patterns are not restricted to individual written letters or individual spoken segments; they apply to the production of the word, phrase, and sentence as a whole.

The term "suprasegmentals" is used interchangeably with prosodic features, nonsegmentals, and rhythm and intonation patterns. The author prefers the expression "rhythm and intonation patterns" because it is a functional description and more easily understood by teachers and clinicians. Also, the word "supra" means above the segmental, or above the consonants, vowels, and syllables. Strictly speaking, this is not true; developmentally, prosody is actually situated below the segmentals. The infant first develops prosody at the preword level, providing a foundation for meaningful spoken language.

Other reasons the author prefers "rhythm and intonation" over "suprasegmentals" is that the implication of "suprasegmentals" is that they are processed primarily through the ear, whereas "rhythm and intonation" include feelings and emotions that are produced by the whole body. "Rhythm and intonation" can be applied to both listening skills and speaking skills. For example, the clinician can assess the child's listening skills for perceiving the sentence "Mama blew a bubble." Does the child demonstrate auditory perception of the speech rhythm by imitating the clinician's model, even though he or she may not produce all the phonemes correctly? Rhythm patterns are also targeted when the mother holds her infant close to her body while she vocalizes. In this case, the infant feels the mother's speech rhythm throughout his or her whole body. With this "whole body" input, the infant will vocalize back, moving his or her body in harmony with the vocal patterns.

The clinician always begins with assessment and treatment of the suprasegmental speech patterns for both children and adults. These patterns provide the foundation for the brain's processing (speech perception) and the production of meaningful speech. In a speech dialogue between two adults, the suprasegmentals (38%) along with body language (55%) provide 93% of the speech dialogue, whereas only 7% is provided by its words and syntax. When toddlers have a speech dialogue with a limited number of words, the suprasegmentals and body language play an even greater role in speech intelligibility.

The low-frequency speech frequencies, below 500 Hz, are optimal for processing speech rhythm and intonation patterns. The body provides input to the brain through movements, vibrotactile speech input from the low frequencies, and proprioceptive feedback. This is why the Speech Strategy for learning should be based on the whole body. The ancient philosophers accurately said, "Nothing is in the brain that is not first in the body senses." So, listening is intimately linked with the motoricity of the child's body. The next section provides examples of suprasegmental assessment.

Voice Quality

Voice quality is a perceptually-based measure that is determined by the physical activity of the laryngeal structures, adequacy of breath support, movement of the articulators, and the underlying emotions and intentions that drive the spoken production. Voice quality contributes to a speaker's social identity and is critical to his or her social acceptance. For example, to fit in among peers, children must be intelligible and use similar dialect or "way of speaking" in order to share a similar quality of voice. Children with normal hearing quickly learn how to control the underlying systems of vocal production, which include respiration, vocalization, articulation, and overall body tension. They establish control over these systems by monitoring their output through the natural auditory feedback mechanism. In contrast, a child with a severe hearing loss, who does not have access to an auditory feedback system, has difficulty regulating his or her voice quality and speech intelligibility. As a result, voice quality and speech intelligibility are often compromised (Alspaugh, personal communication, 2005).

The parameters of voice quality that affect children with hearing loss include decreased breath control, poor timing of vocalizations, inappropriate variations of loudness, posterior tongue position, hyponasality, and irregular pitch and intonation patterns. These parameters coexist and influence voice quality simultaneously, but for greater clarity, they are discussed separately.

Proprioceptive Memory

A child with normal hearing "hears" spoken language and begins to imitate the sounds and speech rhythms that she or he perceives. The child initially imitates single phonemes, but as fine motor skills develop, the child is able to coarticulate and establish a proprioceptive memory for how speech sounds are produced. A child with a severe hearing loss does not have access to a well-developed auditory feedback system, so he or she is not able to process auditory input or develop the memory span that is necessary for speech production. The Verbotonal Approach provides the child with simultaneous auditory, tactile, and proprioceptive feedback through whole body movements, the binaural headset, and the speech vibrator of the Verbotonal Auditory Training Unit. This multisensory input helps the child develop an awareness of normal speech rhythm and intonation as well as facilitates a closer approximation of the articulators for correct speech production (Alspaugh, personal communication, 2005).

Respiration

Speech breathing is markedly different from breathing at rest (tidal breathing). To adequately prepare for speech, adjustments are made to both the inspiratory and expiratory flow of air. In comparison to tidal breathing, which is smooth and steady, speech breathing is rhythmic and pulsatile. For speech, inhalation is rapid and exhalation is prolonged and controlled, so the speaker can sustain the rhythmic patterns of connected speech. Individuals with hearing loss often do not adjust to these speech breathing patterns, and thus are less able to support speech production with an adequate air supply. As a result, their speech production lacks the appropriate rhythm and intonation patterns that give meaning to speech. Without variability and control of exhaled air, speech productions are mistimed, strength and intensity are decreased, and voice quality is monotonous. All of these contribute to a reduction of speech intelligibility (Alspaugh, personal communication, 2005).

Many of the disruptions of voice quality for speech result from inadequate breath support and breath control. Sufficient air supply and proper breathing patterns need to be established first. The Verbotonal Approach to treatment improves breath support by having children hold their breath (speech pause) in anticipation of the next vocalization. Then, the clinician signals the children to vocalize. Coordination of vocalizations with body movements during exhalation improves overall breath support and timing. When movement stops, so should vocalization; this signals the child to inhale (Alspaugh, personal communication, 2005).

Resonance

"Deaf speech" is characterized by a perceptual difference in speech resonance. This is a result of the inappropriate position of the tongue within the oral cavity and the overall restricted lingual movement. The tongue tends to be positioned posterior in the hypopharynx, excessively increasing both nasal and pharyngeal resonance. This particular voice distortion is often referred to as "cul-de-sac" voice. Decreased lingual mobility also interferes with speech production and articulatory accuracy. Individuals with "deaf speech" often undershoot their articulatory targets because of poor posterior-anterior lingual movement. As a result, "deaf speech" is characterized by articulatory imprecision, with a restricted number of vowels and consonants produced (Alspaugh, personal communication, 2005).

The Verbotonal Approach uses whole body movements to increase awareness of muscular tension, vowel duration, intonational changes, and so on. This results in a greater range of lingual movement, which is necessary to achieve correct production of all 15 vowels and diphthongs (Alspaugh, personal communication, 2005).

Vocal Loudness and Vocal Pitch

Vocal loudness and vocal pitch are closely associated and often confused in "deaf speech." Higher pitch is associated with a louder voice and lower pitch with a quiet voice. Given the close relationship between these speech parameters, it is beneficial to target them simultaneously in treatment. For example, vocal pitch and vocal loudness are targeted together with a body movement (Alspaugh, personal communication, 2005).

Auditory feedback provides immediate information used to regulate the loudness of voice. When there is a breakdown in the auditory feedback loop, regulation of vocal loudness is difficult. "Deaf speech" tends to fluctuate in loudness level; at times the voice is too soft and thus misunderstood, and at other times the voice is excessively loud and tense. In both situations, speech intelligibility is compromised. With the Verbotonal Approach, the child relies on proprioceptive feedback (feeling the speech patterns) to monitor speech production (Alspaugh, personal communication, 2005).

"Deaf speech" is also marked by elevated pitch and reduced intonational patterns. The speaker struggles with making changes and adjustments in tension of the vocal cords. This results in either minimal variation or excessive variation of pitch during speech production. For example, the speaker might have a monotone voice quality (reduced variation), making his or her speech unpleasant and difficult to understand. Without proper pitch variation, speech production will not follow normal rhythm and intonation patterns (Alspaugh, personal communication, 2005).

The Verbotonal clinician uses body movements and vibrotactile speech input to develop normal rhythm and intonation patterns, loudness, and overall voice quality. This input provides the feedback so the child can self-correct and produce speech with a normal voice quality (Alspaugh, personal communication, 2005).

Assessment of Rhythm and Intonation Patterns

To assess the suprasegmentals, The Tennessee Test of Rhythm and Intonation Patterns (T-TRIP) is used; it has one to nine syllables with different rhythms and intonation patterns (Koike & Asp, 1982) (Figure 4–1). For example, test item number 1 is a long, stressed syllable followed by a short, unstressed syllable; whereas item number 2 is a short, unstressed syllable followed by a long, stressed syllable. Koike and Asp (1982) tested normal hearing in three- and five-year-old children with the 25 test items of the T-TRIP. Each child imitated the speech pattern he or she perceived, without the help of any visual cues. The clinician judged their responses as either correct or incorrect. The five-year-old children scored 26% higher (86% vs. 60%) than the three-year-old children. This data suggests that rhythm and intonation pattern perception continues to develop in young children and may not be complete until after five years of age. These findings of 60% and 86% are used as reference data for assessing children with perception and production problems. A child with a score of 86% or above is functionally similar to a typically developing five-year-old. The 86% also suggests that the child has mastered the pattern up to nine syllables. This provides a good foundation for perceiving and producing spoken language. In short, the T-TRIP is used to evaluate a child's ability to perceive and imitate rhythm and intonation patterns without requiring language skills; therefore, it can be used with all age groups, including toddlers.

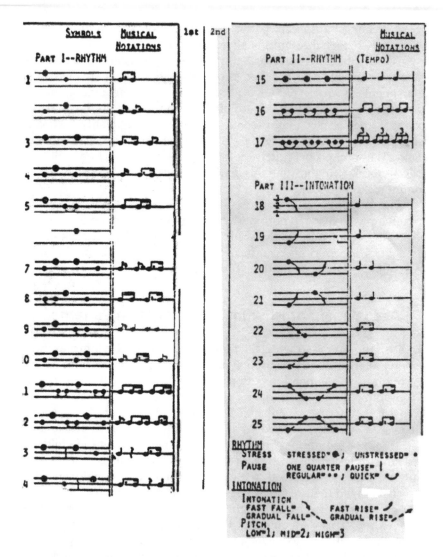

Figure 4–1.   Tennessee Test of Rhythm and Intonation Patterns

For another type of assessment, the Rhythm and Intonation Checklist is used to evaluate each child's ability to perceive and produce speech patterns (Figure 4–2) (Asp, 1985). The left column is speech production with visual cues available, while the right column is auditory perception without visual cues. The clinician begins with the production evaluation because it is the easiest for the child.

Child's Name_____ Years in Program_____

Date of Test_____ Degree of Loss_____

Clinician_____ Testing Conditions_____

I. PRODUCTION (with imitation)

  A. Conditioned to imitate vocalizations
    Yes ( )   No ( )

  B. Duration (long-short)
    1. _____ __
    2. ___ _____
    3. ___ ____ ____
    4. __ __ __
    5. ___ __ ___ __
    6.

  C. Syllables Rate (Elements)
    1. Many-One
    2. One (_____ __ __)
    3. Two (____ ___; __ _ ___;
       ____ __ __; __ __ __ __)
    4. Three ____ ____ ____;
       ____ __ __ ____;
       ____ __ __ ____;
       _ _ __ __ ____;
       _ _ __ _ __ _;
       _ _ ____ __ __)
    5. Four (stressed)
    6. Five (stressed)

  D. Pauses between two or more elements
    Yes ( )   No ( )

  E. Vocal and Intonation Pattern Pitch (circle that which applies)
    1. Voice: high normal low
    2. Changes with one syllable
      a. Upward Inflection
      b. Downward Inflection
    3. Changes within 2 or more syllables
      a. Low to High
      b. High to Low

  F. Vocal Loudness
    1. Loud
    2. Soft
    3. Vary Loudness

  G. Vowels

II. PERCEPTION (with imitation)

  A. Sound awareness-recognizes
    Yes ( )   No ( )

  B. Duration
    1. ___ __
    2. __ ____
    3. ____ ___ ____
    4. __ __ __

  C. Syllables Rate (Elements)
    1. Many - One
    2. One (___ ___ __)
    3. (____ ___; __ __ ___;
       ____ __ __ ____;
       ____ __ __ __;
       __ __ __ __;
       __ __ __ __ __;
       __ __ ___ __ __)
    4. Four (Stressed)
    5. Five (Stressed)

  D. Pauses (different lengths)
    Yes ( )   No ( )

  E. Vocal Pitch and Intonation Patterns
    1. Changes in intonation
      a. Upward Inflection
      b. Downward Inflection
    2. Changes of vocal pitch
      a. Low to High
      b. High to Low

  F. Vocal Loudness
    1. Loud
    2. Soft
    3. Vary Loudness

Figure 4–2. Rhythm and Intonation Checklist

She vocalizes a simple rhythm pattern (e.g., "ah boo bah boo") to assess if the child can imitate some or all of the syllables. Then, she evaluates each speech parameter separately. Can the child imitate a long versus a short speech duration? Can the child imitate a many-to-one speech pattern (e.g., /ba ba ba ba ba (pause) ba/)? To be successful, the child needs to imitate five quick syllables, pause for at least 300 msec, and then imitate one syllable. Next, the clinician evaluates how two quick syllables are perceived and produced relative to longer syllables (e.g./bÙbÙ/—pause—/baaaa baaaa/). The short syllables should be perceived as one beat and the long syllables as two beats. They are rhythm patterns of one perceptual unit and two perceptual units, respectively. Next, the clinician evaluates how the child uses pauses of different length, for example, 200 msec (a normal length pause) versus 100 msec (shorter pause) versus 500 msec (longer pause). Each pause should have a build-up of articulatory tension, followed by a quick release of tension. Next, the clinician evaluates the child's imitation of vocal pitch and intonation patterns. She assesses whether the child's vocal pitch (F_0) is normal, too high or too low (F_0 of 250 Hz is normal for a teenager). Then, she assesses the child's ability to imitate an upward intonation pattern with the vowel /a/ (e.g., 200 Hz to 400 Hz). Later she evaluates an upward intonation pattern followed by a downward pattern in a two-syllable production. Finally, she evaluates the child's vocal loudness. She has the child imitate low-to-high (e.g., 60 dB to 70 dB) and high-to-low (e.g., 70 dB to 60 dB) intensity changes. Can he increase his loudness in stressed syllables and lower it in unstressed syllables?

For a more advanced child, the clinician reduces visual cues and has the child imitate the same rhythm and intonation patterns listed in the right column. If the child can imitate these patterns without visual cues, she has the potential of using auditory feedback to monitor and self-correct her own speech patterns. This ability to self-correct helps the child be an active listener of other's speech patterns as well.

Another test for suprasegmental assessment is the Monosyllable, Trochee, Spondee (MTS) Test in which both suprasegmentals and speech recognition are measured using the same test words. For example, if the test word is "baseball" and the child's response is "softball," the suprasegmentals, placing equal stress on each of the two syllables is correct, but the word recognition is incorrect. However, if the child responds with "baseball," both the suprasegmentals and word recognition are correct. The MTS requires a high language level and word knowledge, which restricts the use of the test.

To assess the child's mean length of utterance and auditory memory, the Speech Rhyme Test (Figure 4–3) is very useful (e.g., /Ah Boo, Bah Boo, Boo Boo, Bah/) (Asp, 1985). These speech rhymes are meaning-

```
I. Preword Rhyme Level
      Ah Boo
      Bah Boo
      Boo Boo
      Bah Boo
II. Consonant and Word-Based Rhymes
      A. Low-Tonality Level: /p/
            Purple Pop
            Purple Pop
            I want more
            Pour Pour Pour
      B. Mid-Tonality Level: /t/
            Tip Toe
            Tip Toe
            Tip Tip Toe
            Toe Toe Tip
      C. High-Tonality Level: /s/
            Shower, Shower
            Take a Shower
            Wash your shoulders
            Take a Shower
```

Figure 4–3. Speech Rhyme Test

ful and fun for a young child. They begin at the preword level (e.g., Ah boo) and then gradually increase in complexity. The child needs a memory length of at least seven syllables to engage in a normal speech dialogue. The Speech Rhyme Test is appropriate for all levels because it includes preword, word, and tonality levels. It is an informal clinical assessment that helps the clinician develop an effective treatment plan, based on the child's auditory memory span. The results of the assessment are used to develop goals and objectives for the child's Individualized Educational Plan (IEP) and to develop an appropriate treatment plan.

Assessment at the Sentence Level

The Syllable and Sentence Test includes a series of sentences that range from simple to complex in structure. The clinician first tests the child's ability to perceive and imitate these sentences. Then, she uses the nonsense syllable /ba/ to imitate an equivalent rhythm pattern to evaluate if the child can effectively imitate the complex rhythm patterns.

Tonality of Speech Sounds

The child's brain uses both the suprasegmental patterns and the segmental tonalities (spectral pitch differences) to perceive speech. Developmentally, the child masters the suprasegmental patterns first; this provides the foundation for the later fine-tuning of the segmental tonalities. The normal rate of speech is 5 syllables and 15 phonemes per second. Once the child is able to process normal rhythm and intonation patterns, he or she can then fine-tune his listening skills and auditory memory in order to perceive the spectral pitch of individual phonemes. For example, the phoneme /s/ is perceived as having a higher pitch than /sh/, and /i/ as having a higher pitch than /a/. This processing of the spectral pitch differences allows the child's brain to auditorily process the individual phonemes at a normal speech rate. The tonality of each segmental speech sound is an important part of the process.

Tonality: Homogeneous Versus Heterogeneous

Why should the clinician use the tonalities instead of the traditional formant frequencies for the treatment plan? In the 1950s, the development of the spectrograph machines allowed researchers to obtain a better insight into the acoustic composition of both vowels and consonants. The spectrograms displayed changes in frequency (Hz), intensity (dB), and duration (msec) of each phoneme in a spoken sentence. It was called "Visible Speech." This acoustic information, while useful in research, did not prove to be an effective tool for speech treatment. The results of using "Visible Speech" with deaf children were very poor. The children could not use this visual representation of speech information to correct their articulation patterns and develop intelligible speech patterns in connected speech. The specific visual information was analytic and could not be transferred into the fast auditory perception necessary in conversational speech.

In contrast, the Verbotonal Approach uses auditory speech perception at the rhythm, intonation, and phoneme level. The clinician uses auditory perception of the specific tonalities to teach the child to perceive them. Tonality (spectral pitch) research began by using an octave filter to separate the speech frequencies to isolate the optimum frequency of each phoneme. First, individual phonemes were recorded by a native talker, then listeners selected the octave filter where perception of the phoneme was the clearest. For example, the vowel /u/ was perceived at a center frequency of 300 Hz, the vowel /a/ at 1000 Hz, and the vowel /i/ at 3000 Hz. For example, consonant /m/ was perceived at a center frequency of 500 Hz, the /d/ at 1250 Hz, and the /s/ at 6000 Hz.

These filter experiments identified the optimum zone for each of the 43 American phonemes (Asp & Guberina, 1981). The results agreed with the tonotopic organization of the cochlea and the brain for phoneme perception. These filter experiments, along with the findings of other related experiments, helped develop a series of spectral pitch comparison experiments among the phonemes. The unfiltered natural speech sounds, with their spectral pitch, were organized on a Tonality Continuum Model that agreed with the Optimal Octave Continuum Model (Asp, 1985). As with the octave filters, these tonality/segmental pitch differences allow the speaker(s) to monitor and self-correct his or her productions and allow the listener(s) to understand the speech output. Typically, the tonalities are naturally and automatically identified both by the speaker and the listener.

Table 4–1 lists the tonalities for the low-, mid-, and high-tonality zones and provides associated words of each (Asp, 1985). For example, low-, mid-, and high-tonality zones correspond to "moo," "cat," and "see," respectively. Normal English-speaking listeners perceive the spectral pitch differences between the word pairs "moo" versus "cat," "moo" versus "see," and "cat" versus "see," and so on naturally. Tonality pitch differences between the individual spoken phonemes are also perceived. For example, there is a pitch difference between the vowels (i.e., /u/ vs. /a/, /u/ vs. /i/, and /a/ vs. /i/) and between the consonants (i.e., /m/ vs. /k/, /m/ vs. /t/, and /t/ vs. /s/). The strategy is that both vowels and consonants are processed along the tonality continuum, (i.e., vowels /u-o-a-e-i/ and consonants /m-n-b-p-g-k-d-dz-t-ts-s/), which ranges from low to high tonality. For assessment, homogeneous tonality is used to evaluate a child's auditory processing in each of the separate zones. This is accomplished by using nonsense syllables, words, or sentences that have vowels and consonants from the same or similar tonality zones. The nonsense syllables /mumu/, /lala/, and /sisi/ are 100% homogeneous because both the vowels and consonants are from the same tonality zone. For words, the homogeneous arrangement of at least 60% of the phonemes is used; for example, the word "teach" has the /t/ and the /tʃ/ from the mid zone and the /i/ from the high zone. This allows a more precise assessment of the child's auditory processing in adjacent tonality zones.

In a spoken syllable, the tonality of the vowels has a greater influence on the child's auditory processing than does the tonality of the consonants, because the vowels carry more acoustic information. The vowel, the nucleus of a syllable, has a greater duration than the consonant(s); therefore, it is a more prominent perceptual feature of the

Table 4–1. Tonality Word Lists

	Low	L-M	Mid	H-M	High
List 1	moon	up	hat	die	seat
	boom	pump	flag	tight	she
	blow	hole	add	raid	thief
	rope	lawn	lot	day	stick
	old	down	fun	red	kiss
List 2	move	nut	rag	lie	crease
	rum	done	ham	height	cheat
	bow	vote	mad	take	tea
	pope	wall	not	gate	six
	no	round	truck	check	fish
List 3	rule	gum	rat	high	cheek
	pool	bug	dad	shine	key
	blown	boat	lamb	tale	east
	mow	all	hot	hate	this
	owe	pound	duck	led	is
List 4	prune	run	crack	kite	teeth
	mood	bump	jack	ice	each
	bowl	roll	had	trade	seek
	roam	law	jar	date	it
	low	plow	love	yet	sit
List 5	noon	blood	cat	hide	eat
	blue	won	rack	sight	tease
	mold	note	tag	face	cheese
	robe	ball	car	rake	itch
	bone	noun	cut	let	chick
List 6	wound	gun	tack	eye	sheet
	broom	bud	hair	tide	ease
	mole	loan	fad	eight	see
	pole	wrong	rock	they	stick
	own	loud	turn	jet	thick

syllable. This is why in treatment we start by targeting the perception and production of vowels in syllables. Also, with the vowel in the medial position, the tonality of the initial consonant has been shown to have a greater affect on auditory perception than the tonality of the same consonant in the final position. Therefore, to select syllables that are homogeneous in tonality, the tonality is similar for the initial consonant and the medial vowel. For example, for the word "move," the /m/ and the /ʊ/ are low tonality, and the /v/ is a low-mid tonality. The homogeneous tonality of the /m/ and /u/ are the most important, with the /v/ having the least importance in tonality perception.

One study compared three homogeneous syllables (initial consonant and medial vowel from the same tonality zone) and six heterogeneous syllables (initial consonant and medial vowel from different tonality zones). Based on the listener's judgment, the experimenter ranked the tonalities of all nine syllables in order from low to high. The final rankings were: /mumu, lulu, mama, susu, lala, sasa, mimi, lili, sisi/. The /mumu, lala, sisi/ are underlined because they are the 100% homogeneous tonality syllables with the initial consonant and the vowel from the same tonality zone. As predicted, the three homogeneous syllables occupied the first (lowest), fifth (middle) and ninth (highest) positions on the continuum. On the other hand, the maximum heterogeneous syllables were /mi/ (lowest consonant and highest vowel) and /su/ (highest consonant and lowest vowel), and they occupied the fourth and seventh positions on the continuum, respectively. From this study, normal listeners were able to perceive differences along the tonality continuum.

Therefore, it is reasonable that the teacher-clinician can use tonality as an accurate way to assess auditory perception in the low-, mid-, and high-tonality zones, for example /mumu, lala, sisi/. In addition, the tonality zones for nonsense syllables, words, and sentences are also useful for specific error analysis (e.g., high error for a mid target), percent correct (e.g., 80% mid-zone vs. 10% high zone), and the developmental order of phonemic progression in children (e.g., "mama" by 2 years of age and "see" by 7 years of age).

Developmental Progression of Tonalities

The developmental progression of phoneme acquisition by children with normal hearing begins with low-tonality consonants (i.e., /p, b, m/) between 18 months and 3 years of age, then progresses to the mid-tonalities (i.e., /t, d, k, g/) between 2½ and 4 years of age, and finally to the high-tonality consonants (i.e., /s, ts, dz, z/) between 3½ and 8 years of age. The vowels are actually attained earlier than the consonants, usually acquired between 6 months to 3 years of age, progressing from the low /u/, to the mid /a/, to the high-tonality, /i/. Although the developmental age and rate varies between vowels and consonants, acquisition of both follows the same pattern of low to mid to high tonalities. Before 18 months of age, prior to phoneme acquisition, most young children rely on "feeling" proprioceptive difference among the phonemes; later they learn to perceive them and distinguish tonality differences.

There is a strong correlation between tonality zones and order of acquisition of both vowels and consonants, which suggests that auditory processing becomes the dominant sensory input for the brain processing of both vowels and consonants. For children, who cannot perceive the tonality differences among the phonemes, their speech patterns will have misarticulation. Severe misarticulation will result in unintelligibility. This tonality developmental model provides a rationale for stimulating and correcting the low tonalities first, the mid tonalities second, and the high tonalities last.

Optimal Octaves

To evaluate auditory processing, the octave filters on the Verbotonal Auditory Training Unit were used to control the speech spectrum of each phoneme in order to determine the optimal octave for each of the 43 American phonemes (Guberina, 1972). Twenty adult listeners with normal hearing selected the octave where each phoneme had its most natural quality (i.e., the vowel /u/ had its "u-ness" and the vowel /i/ had its "i-ness," etc.). From the 20 possible octave bandwidths each with a central frequency, the vowels /u, a, i/ had central frequencies of 250, 1250, and 5000 Hz, respectively; whereas the consonants /p/, /t/, and /s/ had center frequencies of 250, 1600, and 8000 Hz, respectively. The Optimal Octaves Continuum Model corresponds to the Tonality Continuum Model, following the normal phonemic development of typically developing children. It appears that the normal child's brain "tunes" to the tonality of each phoneme, even though there is other acoustic energy across the entire speech spectrum, for example, /a/ at 1000 Hz octave band even though /a/ has energy from 125 Hz to 8000 Hz for a male speaker. This "brain tuning" allows the child to hear and differentiate all 43 phonemes by eight years of age, the same age of acquisition of all the phonemes.

For children with perceptual problems, the clinician selects the optimal octave filter on the Verbotonal Auditory Training Unit to teach and correct the auditory processing of listeners. The optimal octave filter passes only the optimum, or the essence, of the target phoneme, for example, /s/ at 6000 Hz, while attenuating the frequencies of the child's /t/ error (e.g., /ʃ/ at 4000 Hz). This allows the child to hear the tonality difference between the target and the error. This perceived difference promotes self-correction, which generates carryover to conversational speech.

Formant Frequencies: A Comparison

Researchers identified the formant frequencies of vowels and some consonants by an acoustic analysis of each phoneme. Because each phoneme has a unique speech spectrum (frequency response), each formant was identified by its center frequency, which is the frequency (in Hz) with the greatest peak intensity (dB). Each vowel has more than two formants or peak intensities, some of which are similar to the optimal octave. For example, the first formant at 300 Hz for the back vowel /u/ and the corresponding optimal octave of 250 Hz are similar; the first formant of 750 Hz and the second of 1090 Hz for the mid-vowel /a/ are similar to the optimal octave of 1250 Hz; and for the high vowel /i/, the second formant of 2290 Hz and the third of 3010 Hz are similar to the optimal octave of 3000 Hz (Miner & Danhauer, 1977). This suggests a relationship among the vowel production, the acoustic formants, and the person's perception through the optimal octave filter.

To understand how speech perception can be used, the vowel /i/ has some unique qualities. It can be perceived as /i/ with only the optimal octave of 3000 Hz central frequency. However, it can also be perceived as /i/ in a bimodal condition of 250 Hz and 3000 Hz or a broad bandwidth. It appears that the 3000 Hz remains the dominant optimal octave even when the lower frequencies are included. With the unfiltered vowel, /i/, the listener appears to use the high frequency of 3000 Hz because /i/ is higher in pitch than the vowel /a/.

Phonetic Placement: A Comparison

Initially, researchers used a left side-view x-ray to determine the typical articulatory placement of each vowel while the speaker sustained it in one isolated position. An x-ray of the head showed that tongue elevation was the highest for the vowels /i/, /a/, and /u/ in the front, mid, and back positions of the oral cavity, respectively. These x-ray results were used to design the vowel diagram and later for classification of consonants in terms of place (lips to glottis), manner (plosives to glides), voicing (voiceless or voiced), and nasalization (oral or nasal).

This knowledge of vowel and consonant place of articulation is used by most speech pathologists as a phonetic placement treatment strategy. The clinician often points to where the child should place his or her articulators, draws sketches, or uses a mirror for the child to see the correct articulatory position. Although phonetic placement helps children with minor articulation errors, it is not effective in providing a dynamic and lasting impression with severe cases. Phonetic placement is a static model of one position for each phoneme and does not provide information on the dynamics of the ongoing speech that is a function of a series of coarticulations. The acoustic formants and the articulatory placements of the 43 phonemes are useful for understanding how phonemes are produced. However, they are not ideal for effective correction through the child's listening skills. Therefore, the Verbotonal strategy encompasses tonality and the optimal octave continuum for both error analysis and treatment to establish correct perception and production. This is facilitated by the Verbotonal Auditory Training Unit.

Situational Teaching: Pragmatics of Spoken Language

As mentioned previously, the Verbotonal strategy is based on the "Mommy-Baby-Speech-Dialogue," where an attentive, caring mother develops an emotional bond with her infant and uses appropriate speech in meaningful situations. During a given situation or circumstance, the mother draws the infant into a preword speech dialogue, establishing an important interaction with the child. When speech is used in a visually rich interaction, value and meaning are established within the dialogue of spoken language. These initial visual situations provide a context that can be used to teach the meaningful processing and verbalizing of speech. How is this done?

Just as the "Mommy-Baby-Speech-Dialogue" interaction between a mother and her infant facilitates meaningful spoken language, the same speech benefits can be elicited within a child-clinician interaction. To accomplish this, each situation has a unique visual context that provides information that makes speech (preword or word) meaningful. Characters, events, things, circumstances, context, affectivity, and setting are all situational elements that provide a visual context to make speech meaningful. For example, in the case of the normal infant, the characters are usually centered around mama, dada, baby, puppy, kitty, and so forth; the qualities of the characters are big/small, hot/cold, good/bad, and so forth; the events are what the characters do (i.e., eating, drinking, talking, walking, bathing, running, jumping, etc.); and the things are objects used/manipulated by the character (i.e., food, water, juice, ball, car, boat, doll, etc). The circumstances of the situation are what happens minute to minute and why it happens, and the background is where the action and situation occurs (i.e., kitchen, bedroom, playground, bathroom, etc.). The visual context can be manipulated to alter the meaning of the spoken language, but this visual information should remain salient, including those objects, events, and circumstances that are relevant and meaningful to the infant. For the infant to internalize these interactions and recognize spoken language as meaningful, the same simple situations (i.e., eating in the kitchen while having a speech dialogue) are repeated many, many times each day. This repetition provides the redundancy necessary for the infant to understand mommy's speech ("motherese") in the appropriate context in which it is provided. At first, the young infant emotionally responds to mommy's speech by smiling, kissing, or touching. Later, the infant begins to respond with cooing; and in so doing, the mother-infant dialogue progresses from the preword suprasegmental level to the mother-toddler use of word-sentences and sentences as a young child.

These developmental situations can be real or imaginary. At first, the infant understands only real, concrete situations; however, later he or she begins to interpret and use imaginary contexts to role-play the earlier concrete situations. Imagination is an important part in the infant and toddler's development of meaningful speech (spoken language). For instance, as the infant develops these "imaginary" skills, he may only beg for things he or she can see, but will request things that are out of sight, relying on the visual images kept in mind and memory of past experiences to construct his or her request. A normal toddler is able to easily access these memory stores and transition from real to imaginary or imaginary to real situations, understanding the difference between the two.

Most attentive mothers like to read to their infant or toddler. At the beginning, they use simple books adorned mostly with pictures and a limited amount of vocabulary (i.e., Dr. Seuss stories). An effective mother uses affectivity, introducing emotional variations, like an actress, into the story. This brings the story to life for the infant-toddler. She will read the infant's favorite book(s) over and over again as long as the infant enjoys it. This repetition enhances the infant's understanding of the story. For the infant, the affectivity of the mother's presentation, aside from the visual feedback of the pictures, provides meaning. The complexity of the book's content is somewhat irrelevant, because with mommy's high affectivity, the material will be meaningful to the infant because he or she follows the suprasegmentals of mommy's voice and not the individual words. Reading is beneficial and is an important supplement, but it should not take the place of three-dimensional, mother-infant dialogue in real situations. It is within real-life circum-stances that the infant will benefit most in understanding spoken lan-guage and its critical role in everyday interactions.

Segmentals: Error Analysis

An intelligible adult speaker of English uses 43 phonemes, which include 14 vowels, 5 diphthongs, and 24 consonants in conversational speech. Phonetic textbooks provide both the written alphabet letters and the phonetic symbols that represent these speech sounds. To pro-vide effective treatment, the teacher-clinician needs to understand how to use these phonetic symbols. For example, the clinician's speaks the target phoneme /s/, and the child responds with /t/. The target (/s/) and the response of (/t/) are marked with virgules (/ /) around each speech sound. In this example, the child's error was a substitution of the phoneme /t/ for the target phoneme /s/. This provides the differ-ences that commonly exist between the written alphabet letters and phonetic forms; these differences might vary in number and form of the symbols. For example, the word /bit/ has three spoken phones (speech sounds) represented by three phonetic symbols, whereas it has four written alphabetic letters of "beat." Although the number of pho-netic symbols may differ from the number of letters used, both repre-sent the same target word. Practice, experience, and skillful use of phonetic symbols improve the accuracy of the clinician's error analyses and effectiveness of correction procedures.

Some educators, however, do not feel comfortable with phonetic symbols and prefer to use alphabet letters to represent the phonemes. This is acceptable if the educator knows the typical spelling and the exceptions of each phoneme. The most important thing is that the edu-cator can "hear," analyze, and write down the child's error. As long as the difference between phonetic transcription and alphabetic spelling is recognized, and as long as the teacher-clinician is consistent in the method she or he chooses, an effective recording system can be devel-oped using either method.

Optimal Learning Condition

Children who make errors in verbalizing or processing speech obvi-ously are not aware of their errors, or else they would not make them; no one makes errors on purpose. However, older children may become aware of an error(s) because someone calls attention to it. Most of these children do not know how to correct their errors. They feel helpless and frustrated.

Through a systematic analysis of a child's error, the clinician can gather the information necessary in making a correction. Unfortunately, many clinicians are not trained to recognize and use the error(s) to locate the optimal learning condition for the child. However, a trained Verbotonal clinician manipulates the seven speech parameters to present the optimum learning condition to the child through the Verbotonal Auditory Training Unit. The optimum condition is achieved when the child eliminates the error(s) by responding correctly. A successful correction indicates that an optimal learning condition has been established for that particular stage of learning.

The Seven Speech Parameters

To improve the child's speech and efficiently enhance his or her learning, the clinician needs to "hear" the child's speech error(s), analyze it, and modify her own voice to correct the child's error(s). The following seven speech parameters are used for the analysis and modification of the child's speech output: rhythm, intonation, tension, pause, pitch, loudness, and time. These seven parameters occur simultaneously and are perceived globally (together) at all levels of speech; from the pre-word level through meaningful conversational speech. Even though each parameter is interdependent and linked to the other six parameters, it is possible to enhance the child's learning abilities and correct the error(s) by modifying one or more of the parameters individually. This isolated modification system is accomplished by establishing the optimal learning condition for the child. To understand this, each parameter is discussed separately.

Rhythm

Developmentally, rhythm is the most important speech parameter because it provides the foundation for both the processing and verbalizing of speech. How is rhythm processed and interpreted? Essentially, the child's brain has a wide bandwidth, and it "locks-on" to the speech rhythm as one does in tuning a radio. When the locking occurs, the speech signal is clear and there is no static. Without this "locking," speech is a perceptual "blur." For example, an adult listener to a new foreign language, for example, Spanish, has the experience of a perceptual blur. The individual Spanish phonemes, words, and sentences produced by the Spanish speaker cannot be separated by the non-native listener. There is no "locking" possible.

However, with her native language, the "locking on" to the speech rhythm occurs early for a young toddler. If the words or sentences that are presented are too long, the toddler only "locks on" to one part of the speech rhythm. For example, consider "Captain Kangaroo," the main character in an earlier child's television program. His name has five syllables that are spoken naturally in one second, with emphasis or syllable stress on the first and third syllables. Changing the pattern of syllable stress would change the character's name. The same would be true for the meaning of an utterance. These meaningful stress patterns, as well as our rate of production are fundamental to perceiving the speech rhythm correctly.

A particular speech rhythm can be described as fast, slow, or of normal rate (five syllables per second) and is marked by a specific syllable stress pattern. The clinician considers syllable stress in terms of its level of speech to produce it. For example, the level of stress can be primary (more effort and emphasis), secondary (less effort and emphasis), or there may be no apparent stress pattern between syllables. A primary stressed syllable is usually longer in duration (i.e., 300 vs. 150 msec), higher in vocal pitch (i.e., 300 vs. 150 Hz), and louder (70 vs. 60 dB SPL) than less-stressed syllables. In short, more effort changes the duration, vocal pitch, and loudness simultaneously.

A typically developing infant or toddler will successfully process or perceive only those speech rhythms that she has the cognitive capacity to interpret. If the speech signal presented exceeds this capacity, she will perceive a different speech rhythm. Using the earlier example, if her brain's proprioceptive and auditory memory is limited to two syllables per second, then in the example of "Captain Kangaroo," the child's imitation might be /kapnu/. This is a normal-hearing toddler's response to a complex adult rhythm pattern. She processes and repeats only two of the five syllables. When the same child is older and has expanded her auditory memory to a five-syllable pattern, she will perceive and verbalize the complete "Captain Kangaroo" speech rhythm accurately. Even though her speech rhythm is now correct, the child may still demonstrate segmental errors (i.e., /b/k/ and /a/ae/) in her production. The development of normal processing and verbalizing of complex speech rhythm and individual phonemes is not complete until eight years of age for normal-hearing children.

In speech rhythm, words are often classified in terms of their syllable stress pattern, such as monosyllabic (one syllable, i.e., "dog") and two-syllable (i.e., "doggie"). Two-syllable words are further divided into spondaic (two syllables with equal stress, i.e., "hotdog"), trochaic (two syllables with primary stress on the first syllable, i.e., "doggie"), and iambic (two syllables with primary stress on the second syllable, i.e., "above") distinctions.

Recent research has indicated that the first 50 words a child uses follow the same syllable stress pattern. At this stage of learning (typically between 18–24 months), the trochaic syllable stress is the most common. It makes sense that the trochaic syllable stress pattern develops first, because in English, the majority of bisyllabic words are trochaic. However, at a later learning stage, the child can change the syllable stress from the first to the second syllable. This affects both the meaning and the grammatic category of speech. For example, when the noun "object" changes to the verb "object," the phonemic properties are similar, but the meaning of the word is altered. The importance of appropriate syllable stress can be understood by considering a second language learner with a "heavy" accent. Such an individual often processes and verbalizes syllable stress incorrectly, and usually is not understood by a native listener (e.g., 40% intelligible). The heavy accent impedes normal communication because the speech rhythm is different and cannot be processed correctly by the listener. In short, the production of normal speech rhythm patterns, with appropriate syllable stress, is essential for normal speech perception and intelligible speech.

Intonation

The intonation parameter is closely linked to the rhythm parameter and is considered one of the suprasegmental patterns of speech. Intonation patterns include the vocalized pitch changes and the pitch shifts that enhance and affect the meaning of speech and its perception. Vocalized speech is an expression of our affectivity (emotions), and both the infant and the adult rely on emotional changes to communicate a specific meaning. The context of the output, in conjunction with the speaker's emotions, is reflected in the vocal pitch change within the production. Over time, these vocal pitch changes make up the child's intonation patterns.

Our emotions are represented in our speech production by different intonational patterns. The acquisition of these patterns follows a predictable developmental sequence, with the normal infant initially expressing only one or two emotions. By one year of age, the infant's cognitive bank has expanded to include six to nine emotions (happy, sad, angry, content, etc.).

Intonation patterns are divided into two opposing types. The logical or neutral intonation is used in ordinary positive, negative, and interrogative sentences, and affective intonation is used in over 90% of our spoken sentences, expressing our emotions. It is affective intonation that makes speech human and individualized.

To understand the importance of normal speech intonation, one needs to experience a person's neutral voice that has no emotion; this results in a flat intonation (monotone) with no change. To the listener, the flat intonation pattern is difficult to understand and may be interpreted as impolite or rude; the speaker's intended meaning is negatively interpreted. On the other hand, normal speech with good intonation (emotions) makes speech interesting and motivates the listener to interact with the speaker. In short, speech is an expression of our emotions.

The impact of emotions can be illustrated in the word "no," which may have up to eight different meanings, depending on the emotional intonation pattern that is used. The extreme affect is when the word "no" means "yes," the opposite meaning from the spoken word. For example, a young child hears the spoken word "no" often. If said passively, the word "no" can be perceived as "yes," but if said with anger, it means a definite "no," with no other possibilities. The emotional aspect of speech gives an opportunity for the child to be trained in one of the main functions of language; one single word may have several meanings. These meanings depend on the situation, the context, and the speaker's mood.

From an acoustical point of view, intonation patterns are identified by measuring the vocalized fundamental frequency (F_0) and the dependent harmonics and overtones. In expressing emotions, the child's F_0 changes over time, usually within a one- to two-octave range (i.e., the child's mean F_0 of 400 Hz, can range from 200 Hz [minus one octave] to 800 Hz [plus one octave]). The normal speech intonation also includes frequency (pitch) shifts as the child's vocal patterns go "on and off" (i.e., voicing off at 180 Hz, and voicing on at 220 Hz). This is perceived by the listener as a pitch shift and is important in speech processing because speech intonation consists of meaningful pitch shifts and changes over time. For example, an upward intonation goes from a low vocal pitch to a high vocal pitch. These pitch changes and intonation patterns not only influence speech processing, but they also impose physiologic effects on the speaker's body. As vocal pitch increases, body tension also increases in harmony with the tension across the vocal folds (muscular generalization). The tension in the child's body is linked closely to the tension in his or her vocal cords and articulators. It is muscular generalization that provides the direct link between the level of tension in the child's body and the quality of the child's speech production. A high level of tension in the body generalizes to greater tension in the vocal cords, and therefore an increase in vocal pitch.

Pitch: Vocal and Spectral

The pitch parameter is used to analyze both the child's vocal pitch and the spectral pitch (tonality) of the speech sounds. The child's vocal pitch should be natural and pleasant to the listener, resulting in good, appealing vocal quality. All good singers and good speakers have an appealing vocal quality; the listener gets pleasure from hearing it. The natural vocal pitch varies as a function of the age and sex of the speaker. On the average, an adult female has a vocal pitch (fundamental frequency) that is one octave (250 Hz) higher than an adult male (125 Hz). Preschoolers have a vocal pitch that is higher than an adult female. The highest vocal pitch is that of an infant; it can be as high as 800 Hz. By elementary school, both boys and girls have a vocal pitch near that of an adult female. During and after puberty, the vocal pitch of boys lowers to that of an adult male, while girls continue to have a vocal pitch similar to adult females. Of course, there are individual variations in mean vocal pitch within all age groups.

There is a direct relationship between frequency (Hz) and perceived pitch by the listener. The clinician uses pitch judgments of the child's speech in treatment, but uses only frequency (Hz) to understand the relationship among the phonemes.

Even more important is the spectral pitch (tonality) of phonemes, which ranges from low tonality (i.e., /p,b,m/ and /u/) to high tonality (i.e., /s/ and /i/). The spectral pitch is the pitch difference from all the frequencies in a phoneme (i.e., the vowel /i/ is higher in pitch than the vowel /a/). The spectral pitch or tonality corresponds to the tonotopic organization from the cochlea to the brain. The tonality difference allows us to hear the difference among all the speech sounds (phonemes) of American English. Without tonality difference, all speech sounds would sound the same. Children who have unintelligible speech cannot perceive or produce these tonality differences.

Tension

Muscular tension is the dominant physiologic parameter of speech production. It is directly related to the body movements (see Vestibular Strategy, chapter 2) that a clinician uses to stimulate and correct the child's speech errors. It has the advantage over the other parameters because of the direct link between the child's body and articulators, which is muscular generalization.

To understand the physiology of movement, it is important to understand that muscles function in pairs. While one muscle contracts (the agonist), the other muscle relaxes (the antagonist), opposing the movements of the contracting muscle. This physiologic balance between the muscle pairs allows the body limbs to move with precision over time. The precise use of muscular tension over time can be observed when a skilled baseball player hits a 100 m.p.h.-pitched baseball for a home run. The more muscular precision in the baseball swing, the greater the home-run hitter. If, by chance, one set of muscles is overly activated, or is not properly balanced by the antagonist muscle, then the baseball player swings jerkily or late and misses hitting the baseball. The same principle applies to speech production. A normal intelligible speaker can precisely articulate up to 15 speech sounds per second through coarticulation of speech patterns. Some speech sounds have more muscular tension; for example, the vowel /i/ has greater tension than the vowel /a/. This applies to consonants also; for example, (/p/ has more muscular tension than /m/). These tension differences are applied to body movements to indirectly teach a child how to produce the speech rhythm and each speech sound correctly.

From a technical perspective, changes in the physiologic tension can be measured to a certain extent with electromyography (EMG). With surface electrodes attached to the person's skin, the EMG displays voltage increases and decreases over time, reflecting changes in muscle contraction and relaxation, and thus changes in muscle tension.

In a normal speech dialogue, these changes are felt by the listener; there is a close emotional link between the communicating partners. The listener can feel, hear, and see the tension differences in the speaker's voice and body language. The listener actually anticipates the tension changes in the speaker's output because he or she is tuned into the speaker's affectivity. This anticipation is critical for quick and accurate analyses of what is being said. An application of tension was explained in more detail in using body movements for correction.

Loudness

In normal speech dialogue at 3 feet, the speaker uses a loudness level that is most comfortable for himself and for his listener. This is known as the most comfortable loudness (MCL) level, and is on the average 85 dB SPL close to the speaker's mouth and 65 dB SPL at the listener's ear. As a child develops his speech perception, he learns to monitor and adjust his loudness level to be understood by others; for example, he will use more vocal intensity if the distance of the listener is 15 feet, and less intensity if the distance is 3 feet. In normal conversation, at a distance of 3 feet, the child's intensity level (loudness, measured with a sound level meter in dB SPL) varies from less (−10 dB) to more (+10 dB) loudness and vice versa. This normal variation is needed to maximize the listener's understanding. If the child's voice is too loud, too soft, or does not change, it sounds unpleasant to the listener and, therefore, negatively affects the listener's perception. When a speaker has a monotone voice, both his intonation and loudness level do not change.

Each of the 43 American phonemes illustrates the variations of normal intensity of production; each phoneme has a particular intensity (dB) range. For example, the 15 vowels and diphthongs typically have a 7-dB range in intensity (dB), whereas the consonants have a 28-dB range. The vowels have more intensity than the consonants. Although intensity (dB) differences exist, all the phonemes are similar in loudness. For example, a high-tonality consonant /s/ has less overall intensity (in dB) than the low-tonality vowel /u/. However, the consonant /s/ and the vowel /u/ are similar in loudness, because normal-hearing listeners are more sensitive on the high-frequency zone of 2000 to 4000 Hz than the low-frequency zone of 300 to 600 Hz. This heightened sensitivity allows the /s/ consonant to be similar in loudness to the /u/ vowel, which has F1 and F2 below 1000 Hz. Just as interphonemic variations exist, individual phonemes may be produced at a different loudness depending on the context. For example, a stressed syllable increases the loudness of all the phonemes within that syllable, as compared to those in the unstressed syllable(s). In the word /mama/, the first syllable is stressed and sounds louder than the second, unstressed syllable.

Because there is a direct relationship between the intensity (dB) and the loudness perceived by the listener, an increase in intensity increases the perceived loudness. The clinician uses her or his loudness judgment to analyze the child's speaking levels. The intensity level is only important for understanding the relationship among the phonemes.

Time: Duration and Tempo

The duration of individual vowels, consonants, syllables, words, sentences, and so forth are all different. This difference is measured in milliseconds (msec). The rate (tempo) of normal speech is five syllables per second with an average syllable duration of 200 msec. The normal range for vowels is 80 to 150 msec; consonants range from 20 to 80 msec. Vowels demand more time for speech production because they are the nucleus of the syllable, and also because they encounter little resistance from the speech articulators. The "natural" duration (msec) of both vowels and consonants varies in normal connected speech. The duration of some phonemes can be easily varied while others can be varied only slightly. For example, the vowel /ɪ/ in "bit" can have slight variations, whereas the vowel /i/ in "beat" can be produced with a wide variety of variations, either very long or very short. Similarly, the consonant /p/ is restricted in variation change, while the consonant /s/ can be varied from a long to a short duration.

Time can be used to measure changes in duration, speech rate, speech tempo, stress patterns, and so forth. When speech rate and tempo are manipulated, speech processing is affected. For example, a normal adult speech rate may be too fast for an adult with dementia, a child or a person with a hearing impairment, or a second language learner to process it successfully. Most often, in these cases, the listener's impairment results in a shortened proprioceptive and auditory memory span that is not sufficient for processing rapid speech. A sensitive speaker adjusts his or her speech tempo and language content to match the listener's ability so that a successful and effective interaction is maintained.

Timing is a developmental factor in the child's speech. For instance, in the case of "choo choo train," the child may first say "oo oo ain." The absence of consonants is replaced by the lengthening of the three vowels. The same phenomenon is produced by consonants appearing between two vowels (intervocalic). Take the word "coffee." The young child will say first "o ee" then "co ee," but even in this second step a certain lengthening of "ee" is given to replace the absence of /f/. This indicates that the child has to expand his perceptual skills to perceive all the phonemes in the utterance. The process is all part of his normal perceptual development.

Pause

Pause is the physiologic stopping or freezing of the vocal and articulatory movements for brief periods of time (i.e., 200 msec). Each pause occurs with an increase in physiologic tension to "stop, hold, or freeze" the voicing and articulation to highlight or emphasize a particular meaning. For example, the written sentence, "I cannot go out because it is raining," is usually spoken as, "I can't go out, cause it's raining." A long pause (200 to 500 msec), with an increase in physiologic tension and vocal pitch, takes the place of the conjunction "because" and it achieves a more emphatic meaning.

A pause parameter can also occur within words (i.e., "keep"). There is a natural pause between the end of the vowel /i/ and the onset and release of the final consonant /p/. Pauses are the "off-time" in speech rhythm that highlight the "on-time." Gifted oral speakers keep the listeners interested by using pause to emphasize meaning and give the audience a chance to process what was said. For instance, an effective speaker would say, "It's appalling to see the scourging situation in which these poor people have to live!" The stronger the accent and the longer the pause that follows "It's," the more the listener pays attention and understands the intended meaning of what was said. Effective pause is a powerful tool in providing meaningful information to the listener and is important for maintaining normal speech rhythms.

Initially, the pause in speech is felt by the infant-toddler, but later when the listening becomes the dominant parameter, the child is able to auditorily process pauses, even though there is no acoustic energy. The infant and toddler can also use pause at the preword level, carrying the same important meaning as at the word/phoneme level, just explained. The clinician, therefore, uses pause to enhance both analyses and correction of the child's error.

In summary, the teacher-clinician can use these seven speech parameters to analyze and correct the child's errors and modify the next stimulus in order to provide an optimal learning condition. She uses her auditory perception of each parameter, for example, pitch and loudness, not frequency and intensity. Her perceptual skills are critical for helping the child develop normally. She works through all the senses of the body in addition to the ear to develop normal brain processing of speech.

Error Analysis

To be effective, the clinician uses an error analysis strategy within a stimulus-response paradigm that depends on the understanding and manipulation of the seven speech parameters. The seven parameters help the clinician to hear and analyze the young child's error(s), and then implement the appropriate speech modification of the next stimulus. The goal is to achieve a correct response from the child. Her speech modification is based on the child's error. This strategy provides a model for correcting the child's specific production error, but it also sets up a real phonologic dialogue between the child and the clinician.

Stimulus-Response Paradigm

The stimulus-response paradigm always begins with the correction of speech rhythm and intonation, the foundation of spoken language. For example, in the first stage of targeting speech rhythm, the child should vocalize many syllables quickly, then pause and vocalize only one syllable (i.e., /mamamamamama (pause) ma/). The clinician uses speech modification, body movements and vibrotactile input from the Verbotonal Auditory Training Unit to help the child feel the "many-to-one" speech rhythm. Once this is learned, the child can control and verbalize single syllables, repressing the urge to produce many syllables. Later, the child will expand his or her two-syllable production to a trochaic syllable stress pattern (i.e., /mama/).

An example of the clinician's error analysis would be:

> The clinician says /mama/, and the child responds with /baba/. Her error analysis indicated that the child's speech rhythm, intonation, and vowels were correct, but there was a segmental error, /b/ for /m/ substitution. The child's /b/ is more tense than the clinician's target /m/. To implement the optimum learning condition for the child, the clinician decreases her tension on the next /mama/ stimulation. If, by chance, the child did not correct the error, the clinician's next stimulus moves the consonant /m/ to the final position where there is even less tension (i.e., /am/). If the child imitates it correctly, then the clinician then transfers the less tense production of the final /m/ to the initial position. She has to be skillful for the transfer of tension. If the child imitates the target correctly, the clinician had created the optimum learning condition through a series of speech modifications, using different degrees of tension.

The clinician's speech modification usually results in the correction; however, if it does not, the clinician adds a less tense corrective body movement to reduce the child's excessive tension in the initial position. The clinician's refined use of the degree of tension is related to her ability to alter her affectivity (emotions) in her speech modifications. Another treatment tool is the optimal octave filter of 800 Hz, set at a low intensity (dB) to emphasize the optimal frequency of the /m/ consonant. The optimal filter serves to eliminate the frequencies of the child's error. This error analysis strategy, using the seven speech parameters, helps the child hear his or her error and self-correct it. The child becomes a more competent and confident listener. He or she has "fine-tuned" listening skills to monitor his or her speech and that of others. This is the basis of precise listening skills for correcting speech errors.

Permanent Errors

In contrast, some clinicians repeat the same target stimulus several times with the assumption that the "normal target" will result in the child's self-correction. With children who have a severe communication disorder, this does not happen. The clinician may even present the target in a louder and louder voice, and overarticulate it, but to no avail. If the clinician does not use error analysis, the target repetition, without a successful correction, makes the child's error permanent, often becoming a habit and hindering the child's normal development. In short, practice makes permanent but it does not necessarily make the child's production perfect or correct. The key to correcting the speech errors is the Verbotonal clinician's ability to analyze the child's errors and teach the child to successfully self-correct him- or herself. So, if practice does not make it perfect, the Verbotonal clinician must use an effective strategy to correct the child's errors.

Treatment

Situational Teaching

To maximize learning for children with communication disorders, situations are created to teach meaningful pragmatic skills to the infant, toddler, or child, either individually or in small groups. The clinician uses short, meaningful stories that draw the infant, toddler, or young child into the situation. As the young child becomes more interested, he or she will want to act out his or her role from memory. Soon, all the children will want to play a part in the story, setting up a stagelike performance. This active role-play and interaction maximizes the child's memory for a functional use of the pragmatics of spoken language, and "gives them a meaningful context in which to put their newly learned concepts."

An example with a group of children follows:

Initially, the clinician uses a meaningful Fisher-Price toy or a soft-stuffed, doll-like person for each character, for example, the mommy character (mama) has to be meaningful to the infant. The same toy-character pair is used each time so that the infant-toddler can identify the toy person as "mama" with no confusion. There are several levels of complexity of this situational role-play. Functional words such as "mama" and "dada" are chosen for Level 1. The characters have a simple dialogue with four to six scenes in the story. The dialogue could be: "Hi, Mama," "Hi, Baby," "Let's go for a walk," "Where's dada," "Let's walk with dada," "Walk-walk-walk-walk." Later, new characters may be added (i.e., kitty, puppy, etc.) to the story. The child is only an interested observer. Level 2 would begin when the child is drawn into the story, and actively participates as one of the characters. Level 2 continues until all the children are part of the story and are able to remember and verbalize what each character says. In Level 3, all the dialogue between the characters is from memory because each child has internalized the story. The carryover is when each child uses the story in imaginary situations of everyday play, when incidental learning is most effective. Finally, at Level 4 (for older children), the clinician writes out the same situational stories and vocabulary to teach reading and writing. The children learn to read and write the same dialogue that was used in the previous situations. The increased complexity of linguistic skills that are required to successfully meet the demands of the task at Level 4 prepares the child for mainstreaming into the regular school classrooms with little or no accommodations.

Didactic to Incidental Learning

As a general rule, the more severe the communication disorder, the more intense the didactic treatment needs to be, especially during the critical developmental stages of the infant and toddler. For example, a child with a profound hearing impairment (i.e., +90 dB HTL), with limited residual hearing, needs intensive everyday didactic treatment for three or more years. A child with a severe hearing impairment, (i.e., 70 dB HTL) needs only one to two years of intensive treatment to be an effective hearing aid(s) user. A child with a cochlear implant will usually make faster progress than a child with a hearing aid(s). Determining the appropriate level of treatment is important for the child's success in the school's mainstreaming program.

For children with a cochlear implant, some educators rely mostly on incidental learning, because the implant-aided pure-tone thresholds are near or within normal audiometric limits (25 dB HTL). The educator may assume that the child has normal hearing because of the 25 dB thresholds. The decision to use only incidental learning in the early stages of the child's development may create a problem later if the child does not have the foundation of rhythm and intonation speech patterns. Incidental learning should be used in conjunction with other instructional strategies. The author recommends beginning with an effective didactic correction strategy to set the stage for the ongoing incidental learning that the child will carry over to his natural environment. The self-correction by the child maximizes the incidental learning, thus promoting successful generalization of the skills learned in the treatment to everyday, natural environments. The appropriate balance between didactic and incidental learning is needed for the child to develop naturally. The multidisciplinary team is responsible for watching this closely to determine an appropriate Individual Education Plan (IEP) for each child.

References

Asp, C. W. (1985). The Verbotonal method for management of young hearing impaired children. *Ear and Hearing*, 6(1), 39–42.

Asp, C. W., & Guberina, P. (1981). *Verbotonal method for rehabilitating people with communication problems.* New York, NY: World Rehabilitation Fund, Inc.

Guberina, P. (1972). *The correlation between sensitivity of the vestibular system, and hearing and speech in verbotonal rehabilitation* (Appendix 6, pp. 256–260). Washington, DC: Office of Vocational Rehabilitation, Department of Health, Education, and Welfare.

Kim, Y., & Asp, C. W. (2002). Low frequency perception of rhythm and intonation speech patterns by normal hearing adults. *Korean Journal of Speech Sciences*, 9(1), 9–16.

Koike, K., & Asp, C. W. (1982). Tennessee test of rhythm and intonation patterns. *Journal of Speech and Hearing Disorders*, 46, 81–87.

Miner, R., & Danhauer, J. (1977). Relationship between formant frequencies and optimal octaves in vowel perception. *American Audiology Society*, 2, 163–168.

CHAPTER
5

Second Language Strategy: Auditory-Based

Bilingualism

The Easiest Way to Speak a Second Language

First, let us consider an ideal learning situation. While American parents are living in Spain, they enroll their preschooler in a daycare class, which has 15 preschoolers who speak Spanish as their native language. The class meets daily, 8 AM to 5 PM, and the class is based on developmentally appropriate play, social activities, and spoken language. There is no written language used for preschoolers. The daycare teacher has lived in Spain all her life, and speaks only Spanish to her class.

The Expected Results of an American Preschooler

At the end of three months or 480 daycare hours (40 × 12 weeks), plus after-class interactions in a Spanish speaking culture, the American preschooler will fluently speak Spanish at the same level as his Spanish-speaking preschool peers. The American preschooler will sound like a native Spanish preschooler and will be accepted socially if his Spanish dialect is the same as his peers.

If his American parents are also fluent in Spanish and speak only Spanish to the preschooler at home, the child will sound even more native. However, if the parents do not speak Spanish or speak a "broken" Spanish, the result will still be excellent, as long as the preschooler can interact with Spanish speaking people and/or watch Spanish television in the evenings and on weekends. The preschooler is truly bilingual at this point, fluent in both English and Spanish.

An Ideal Situation

The situation needs to be analyzed on both a theoretical and practical basis. If we understand why this is successful, we can design and implement successful second-language programs. Similar programs can also be implemented to help children with a communication disorder to learn their native language.

First, the age of the preschooler is optimal because of the neuroplasticity of the child's brain (i.e., the ability to learn and remember new things). Learning "old" information does not interfere with the learning of "new" information. In short, the child's native "tongue" (brain perception from the vestibular system) does not interfere with the child's "ear" (brain perception from the cochlea). Even though the American preschooler is fluent in speaking his native American language, the motor habits of his tongue (articulators) while speaking English phonemes do not interfere with learning the tongue (articulatory) movements and listening to the Spanish phonemes.

The major difference is that the American preschooler was able to learn a new set of rhythm, intonation, accent, dialect, and body language patterns. Even though the Spanish and English patterns are different, the child was able to internalize the new motor pattern of Spanish and this became rapidly automatic in daily use. At this point, he or she sounds like a Spaniard. The learning and internalization of the Spanish phonemes and syllabic patterns now are possible because the preschooler is no longer "hard-of-hearing" for the phonemes and syllabic patterns of the second language. There is in a sense a "release from masking" (i.e., American [the native language] motor speech patterns do not interfere with Spanish [the foreign language] motor patterns) and the child can "hear" (or, better said, "feel") the fine differences among Spanish phonemes and prosody. To reduce or eliminate the negative effect of the native language on the foreign language is the major challenge of teaching a second language.

From a neurologic point-of-view, the American preschooler has not developed a dominant right ear (left hemisphere) for speaking his American language. Both hemispheres are independently active in his brain perception. However, if he were a teenager, his corpus callosum would be fully myelinated, which has both hemispheres functioning as one hemisphere in learning a second language.

The Perceptual Factors That Affect Learning

Movement and Memory

The American preschooler is always moving (vestibular perception) while speaking (voicing) in the daily social play with Spanish preschoolers. This movement enhances the child's memory patterns. His or her brain is programmed for the rhythm and intonation of Spanish.

Emotional Intelligence (EI) or Quotient (EQ) of Spanish

All the play situations include affect, drama, surprise, imagination, and spontaneous emotions that help develop the preschooler's emotional intelligence (EI) for Spanish. The child's range of emotions is reflected in the child's different intonation patterns. Changes in intonation patterns change the meaning. For example, the word "no" spoken with a variety of emotions alters the meaning of the word so it can have multiple (four to ten) meanings. It can even mean "yes," the opposite of "no," if "no" is said with the appropriate emotions and context. With an average of 10 meanings per word, the child now could have 250 meanings for only 25 words!

Rhythm and Accent Speech Patterns

The brain's ability to perceive the speech rhythms of Spanish occurs when the child "feels" the speech rhythms through vestibular perception. This is what may be called "body perception." After the speech rhythms are internalized in memory, the child can recall different patterns by only listening. Speech rhythms and rhymes feel and sound pleasant to his or her brain. Good rhythm perception allows the child to anticipate the rhythm patterns of the speaker. In short, it enables the preschooler to anticipate what a Spanish preschooler will say and also hear rapidly with ease and pleasure.

Social Situations in Learning

The social situations (context) in the daycare program are constantly changing from moment to moment and minute to minute. The meaning of the word or sentence is determined by the situation. Each situation is different. The preschooler attained the memory of the Spanish words from the social situations. The situation can be either real or imaginary. Preschoolers can switch from real to imaginary or vice versa and know the difference. Play and imagination are important in emotional intelligence (EI) for learning the subtleties of the Spanish language.

The situation also requires role playing, whereby, the preschoolers assume the role of different characters (i.e., mommy, daddy, baby, puppy, etc.) in the same situation. Playing the role of others allows the preschooler to learn the language of the other speakers and remember it.

Auditory-Visual (AV) of Situations

Both the auditory and the visual senses are important in learning. The visual input is dominant at first, because the preschooler can see and understand the meaning through the actions of the social situation. As the child's receptive language grows quickly, he or she can understand the meaning from a global point of view. However, as the expressive language grows, the auditory becomes the dominant modality for learning to hear and speak Spanish.

Hearing the Error

All preschoolers make many segmental (speech sound) errors in the early stages of learning Spanish. The developmental norms show that segmental errors decrease and continue until eight years of age. The child learns tonotopically, beginning the mastery of low tonality and working toward high tonality (i.e., /b/ to /s/). This development is based on auditory perception. That is why many early words are made of low frequencies (i.e., papa, mama, baby, yum yum, bow wow).

The child will make some errors in speech rhythm if the spoken sentence is longer than his or her proprioceptive and auditory memory. For example, a seven-syllable utterance is spoken but the child only has enough memory for three syllables. The child will repeat back only the three syllables but keep the rhythmic pattern. However, the prosodic features are already standard. The prosodic frame can be easily recognized. By eight years of age, the child's memory is greater than seven syllables, and the child can process longer sentences with some more complex structures of a language.

Within the first year of life, the child perceives the emotions of the speech of his parents and friends. By the age of two, the child has developed many emotions and perceives all the emotions through the speaker's intonation pattern. The child rarely makes an error in the perception of emotions. To make an error of an emotion is to not understand what is said.

The preschooler can perceive (hear) these errors and gradually correct them, first, at the rhythm and intonation level and, later, at the phoneme level. Preschoolers can perceive and correct their speech errors because they can "hear" the error(s). However, adults in the same social situations cannot "hear" their errors so well. As a result, without any negligence on their part, they make their errors permanent and will always keep the wrong accent patterns. Typically, adults will never be accepted as native Spanish speakers unless they receive an intensive Structuro-Global-Auditory-Visual (SGAV) program or its equivalent.

Dreaming in Spanish

The preschooler will begin dreaming in Spanish during the intensive three-month daycare program. This dreaming, with rapid eye movements (REM), "refreshes" the brain and helps the preschooler to remember the new Spanish language. This allows the child's perception to be internalized and automatic. It is analogous to learning to swim.

The Structuro-Global-Auditory-Visual (SGAV) Protocol

The SGAV protocol originated with Professor Guberina (1972) was improved by Professor Roberge to develop good spoken second language skills for adults and older children. It also is effective with preschoolers. The theoretical basis of SGAV is based on the following strategies.

Theoretical Basis for SGAV Method

Learning to speak a second language is easier and more successful for children under five years of age. These children can be placed in a social environment with other children who speak the second language (i.e., daycare program), and they will learn to speak the second language with the same rhythm, intonation patterns, accent, and body language as the children who are native speakers. As explained earlier, while in Spain an American English speaking child preschooler attends a Spanish preschool program daily. The English-speaking child can then learn the spoken language with the correct accent without any interference from adults. These young children learn the rhythm and intonation patterns of the second language before they learn the individual phonemes. In addition, they learn in situations that have meaning from which they are able to abstract meaning of the spoken language due to the redundancy of the situations. No one tells them the meaning of each individual word or sentence.

Between 8 and 12 years of age, second language learning in a similar situation is more difficult because the first language impedes the learning of the second language. However, rhythm, intonation, and accent are better learned by the 4- to 12-year-old than by an adult. After approximately 13 years of age, when the child has passed through puberty, he or she already is physiologically an adult due to the maturation of his brain. These neuronal differences result in difficulty learning the rhythm, intonation, and accent of the second language. Most lay observers and some professionals think that the difficulty occurs with the individual phonemes of the second language. However, the auditory processing and the learning of the rhythm, intonation, and the accent are the true main issue.

At an adult age, the corpus callosum has completely myelinated, connecting the two hemispheres. In most cases, the left hemisphere (right ear) becomes the dominant hemisphere for the first language. Now, the native "tongue" interferes and masks the listening of the "ear" for the second language. In other words, the rhythm and intonation patterns of the first language interfere (mask) and block the learning of the second language. The learner cannot hear clearly the phonemes of the second language or its accent patterns because of the masking and cannot relate it to the meaning because the situations are not clearly heard.

Public school systems and universities have not been successful in teaching spoken language and listening skills to the level where the students develop the same rhythm, intonation, and dialect of the first language. Most of their students are not accepted as native speakers in a foreign country. Until the student is accepted as a native speaker in a second language, he or she has not internalized the essence of the language. Most of these programs concentrate on grammar rules or dictionary usage of vocabulary and conjugating of verbs to understand the written language. Written language is a separate entity from the spoken language. This is a rote memory process that is not retained by the students. After two years away from the language, students typically forget most of what they learned. It is like studying a dictionary and not remembering the meaning of words without a daily functional use of those meanings.

Another problem in this learning strategy is the language listening labs that have been set up in universities and some public schools for learning how to speak the language. The flaw in this particular strategy is that a broadband signal from a tape is presented to the second-language learner from which they write down the meaning and attempt to imitate what they hear. Because their native tongue interferes with their ear, they are unable to hear the second language clearly and leisurely. As a result students will continue to make errors in spoken language and will have no idea that any errors occurred. The reason for unidentified errors is because they cannot hear the differences between what they hear on the tape and what they say. Even if they do hear the differences, they do not know how to self-correct the error. However, if the same students were in a SGAV class with at least 90 hours of intensive stimulation and correction through spoken language listening, they would be able to go to the listening lab and hear some external differences on the audiotape. This allows students to hear their errors when they produce a word in a sentence and to self-correct. The key is the ability to self-correct.

Another problem is that most of the second-language teachers are not native speakers of the language they teach. That is especially true in high school foreign language programs. However, in universities, the instructors are mostly native speakers. Unfortunately, many times university instructors do not have a strategy for building new patterns of rhythm and intonation and listening skills for the second language. Their teaching strategy does not follow the ideal learning situation explained in this chapter.

SGAV Teaching Strategy

The structuro-global-auditory-visual method uses filmstrips with audiotapes or just videotapes for teaching in natural situations for the students to learn the meaning of spoken language. Within each lesson for each language, there are 10 to 20 visual pictures using questions, answers, reactions, affective comments, and so forth. The lesson is a step toward a progression in conversational skills, from easy to difficult. For example, a first lesson in English as a second language might be . . . Line 1: Hello, John. Line 2: How are you? Line 3: I am fine, thank you. Line 4: Dorothy, this is John. Line 5: He is my friend. Line 6: I am so pleased to meet you. Line 7: I am Dorothy. Line 7: Dorothy is my wife. Line 8: Are you visiting New York? Line 9: Yes, I am visiting New York. Line 10: Is this your house? Line 11: Yes, this is my house. Line 12: Would you like to come in? Line 13: Yes, I would like to come in. Line 14: It is getting late, good night. Line 15: See you later. This is an example of a situation that tells a story and has a beginning and an end.

There are three characters: John, Dorothy, and the speaker. This situation with questions, answers, and so forth makes one lesson. Fifteen lessons or situations comprise stage 1 of that language. During the early learning phase of up to 60 hours of listening, no reading or writing of the spoken language occurs. However, after the 60 hours, the written words and sentences are used with the beginning lessons so that the students can learn to read and write the spoken words that are used in these conversational situations.

As with the preschoolers, movements should be used to enhance the drama, affect emotions, whole body, and gestures. This will increase the emotional intelligence in mastering the second language. The specifics of these movements are explained in a subsequent chapter.

The Auditory Basis of SGAV

The Verbotonal Auditory Training Unit for a classroom is a four-channel training unit that includes: (1) a broad bandwidth from 20 to 20,000 Hz, (2) 300 Hz low-pass, (3) 3000 Hz high-pass, and (4) a restricted band from 300 to 3000 Hz (similar to the telephone). Each of these four channels is operated by an illuminated push button that is user-friendly. Channel 1 (broad bandwidth) is used for introducing the filmstrips and audiotapes to understand the meaning of the 15 pictures with questions and answers in lesson 1. However, to break the effect of the first language on the second language, the next stage is imitation with the audiotape through channel 2, a 300 Hz low-pass filter. The 300 low-pass filter preserves the rhythm and intonation of the second language but eliminates the intelligibility of it. Therefore, the listeners have an easier time of imitating the new rhythm and intonation of the second language. During this stage, the teacher needs to identify the errors of each of the classroom members and correct them immediately after they make their imitation. The audiotapes provide a model for the standard from the second language; the teacher imitates the model correctly for the students. Upon successive imitation with corrections, the students will hear the difference between the tape, the teacher, and each student's imitation. This will allow them to learn the correction of errors through listening. The key to success in this method is the teacher's ability to modify the next stimulus for the correction. Along with body movements or gestures, the teacher needs to understand the seven perceptual parameters identified earlier in this text and use them effectively in the correction within the stimulus-response framework. Through understanding of these parameters, the early stages of rhythm and intonation correction with the 300 Hz low-pass channel can be accomplished. Then, the training unit can be changed to a more advanced level.

The second level is bimodal when channel 3, the 3000 Hz low-pass filter, is added to channel 2, the 300 Hz high-pass filter. The additional speech energy increases speech intelligibility. However, it does not pass the 300 to 3000 Hz range, which includes the phonemes of the first language that interfere with the listening. Once the second stage of bimodal is achieved then the teacher changes to channel 4, the 300 to 3000 Hz range, for listening to the phonemes of the second language. Channel 4 is similar to the range of the telephone system. After the 300 to 3000 Hz bandwidth is mastered with no interference, the broadband is used as an everyday listening situation in spoken language.

SGAV: Individual Correction with Optimal Octaves

The Verbotonal Auditory Training Unit is used for individual sessions with students who are having difficulty keeping up with other class members. After about 20 hours of classwork, there is a separation among classmates. Most students do very well; however, a few students are not able to hear the differences in the rhythm and intonation patterns or the phonemes. The optimal octaves identified earlier for each language are used for the correction. For example, to correct the "s" sound in the second language, the octave filter is set for the center frequency of 6000 Hz under headsets. Using a microphone, the teacher corrects the students in listening for the "s" sound of the second language. The filter does two things: (1) it passes the optimal frequencies for the perception of "s" in that language, and (2) it filters out or attenuates the frequencies that are used in the substitution error. This way the student learns to hear the phoneme clearly and to distinguish it from other phonemes in adjacent frequency zones.

Another example that is more difficult to correct is the American vowel /ae/, like in the words "cat, sat, apples." For this correction, the optimal octave of 1600 Hz center frequency is set as the teacher says /ae/. If the error is the vowel /a/, the teacher uses more tension in producing /ae/ or uses the filters above to increase the chances of a correction to the vowel, in the case of Spanish (Mexican, Puerto Ricans, etc.), Italian, or Arabic-speaking people. On the other hand, if the pronunciation is /e/ (in the case of French, Polish, Chinese, and Russian speakers), the teacher could use relaxation on the channel immediately lower than 1600 Hz. The combinations of the optimal octaves and the choice of the right tension provide an optimal condition for the correction.

This individual treatment with the Verbotonal Auditory Training Unit along with the modification of one or more parameters is critical in the early stages of learning and keeps each student on the same level as other members of the class. After a student hears the phoneme in the filtered situation, his or her brain is tuned to the frequency zone (optimal octaves) of that phoneme. As a result, when they hear broad bandwidth of an everyday life situation, the brain is still attuned to the frequency zone of the phoneme. This is an advanced level of listening and results in carryover to real-life situations.

Group Correction and Nursery Rhymes

Group Correction

When the SGAV teaching is done with a group of students, the weak students hear the errors and corrections of the better students. Then they are able to self-correct themselves naturally. Although the better students may not be as good as the teacher who serves as the model for listening, the weak students can hear the differences between the model and the better students. Older students are also helped in this way. Even if they do not self-correct completely, they at least show some improvement.

Nursery Rhymes

A second way is the use of nursery rhymes where speech rhythm is the foundation of listening and speaking correctly. But what is speech rhythm? In order to teach the rhythmic patterns of a second language, the teacher needs (a) a fixed and regular rhythmic pattern of accents for each line of the nursery rhyme (2, 3, or 4 accents); (b) repetitions of phonemes, syllables, and rhymes; (c) usually a four-line pattern is better; and (d) four to eight syllables for each line (Roberge, personal communication, 2001).

For example:

Number of syllables		Number of accentuated syllables
5	*Rain, rain, go away*	4
7	*Come again another day*	4
5	*Rain, rain, go away*	4
6	*Little Johnny wants to play.*	4

This rhyme contains four lines, with "rain" repeated four times, four accents for each line, and the rhymes are of the diphthong /ei/ repeated four times. Another example is:

Number of syllables		Number of accentuated syllables
4	*Five little monkeys*	3
5	*Jumping on the bed*	3
3	*One fell off*	3
4	*And bumped his head*	3
6	*Mama called the doctor*	3
5	*And the doctor said*	3
5	*"No more little monkeys*	3
5	*Jumping on that bed"*	3

Then this is repeated with:

Four little monkeys . . .

Then:

Three little monkeys . . .

Etc.

Speech rhythm exists also when the teacher uses repetitions. For example:

Number of syllables		Number of accentuated syllables
4	*This is my <u>house</u>.*	2
7	*These are the <u>ears</u> of my house.*	3
7	*This is the <u>mouth</u> of my house.*	3
7	*This is the <u>nose</u> of my house.*	3
7	*These are the <u>eyes</u> of my house.*	3
8	*These are the <u>eyebrows</u> of my house.*	3
7	*This is the <u>hair</u> of my house.*	3
7	*These are the <u>arms</u> of my house.*	3
7	*These are the <u>hands</u> of my house.*	3
4	*<u>Hello</u>, my house!*	2

If the rhythm of the nursery rhyme is properly learned, its individual sounds are naturally corrected as the given rhythmic frame is one that allows only the phonemes of the language in question and no others. This may be confusing for some readers, but the "proof is in the pudding" (i.e., it works). Another rhythm would allow other types of phonemes, syllables, or accents. Correct phonemes spring from their well.

Pictures to illustrate these nursery rhymes help a lot. They may serve:

- To facilitate the memorization and reproduction

- For the understanding of the meaning. By so doing, translation is avoided and learner participation is activated

- For different games

- For the feeling of different rhythmic patterns

- And, finally, to give self-confidence to the learner

As a result, the learner is pulled into the rhythmic pattern of the nursery rhyme. He cannot oppose or resist. He is like somebody who goes to a disco. At first, he refuses to dance but after five minutes of listening to the rhythm of the music, he feels compelled to join in. If he did not, his body would need excessive energy to resist or to leave the disco.

SGAV: Order of Teaching the Audiovisual Portion

Using the Verbotonal Auditory Training Unit and the audiovisual tapes and filmstrips, the teacher begins the first stage of preparation by assuming the mood (affect) of the second language. This can be done in a very global way through a total immersion into the second language. With lesson 1, the broadband frequency response is always used. The teacher goes through each of the 15 questions and answers and has the students discuss the meaning of that language. After they have an overall idea of the second language, the teacher emphasizes the second language for each of them. No dictionaries or written references are allowed in class.

Stage 2 is the presentation under the 300 Hz low-pass filter for the imitation of the rhythm and intonation patterns. The teacher continues on with these lessons until the class can imitate the rhythm and intonation of the second language in all 15 questions and answers. This is repeated with the bimodal (lows and highs) presentation, the telephone response, and finally the broadband situation. This is a progression of listening skills from the very difficult rhythm and intonation patterns to the fine-tuning of individual phonemes with the meanings from the situations.

Stage 3 goes from the imitation stage to the acting (role-playing) stage of the situation. For example, one student becomes Dorothy, another one, John, and one student, the speaker. Now without any help from the audiovisual aids, the student begins to role-play the entire dialogue from lesson 1. This role-playing tests their memory and ability to understand situations. The teacher corrects individual things said by the students (i.e., Hello, John.). If it is not said correctly, the teacher does the correction immediately and requires the student to imitate again. However, the intent of the role-playing is for the students to memorize and to be spontaneous in acting out this lesson as if it were a play in theater. This allows each individual student and class member to emotionally live in the situations of the second language. Through the emotional attachment of living each lesson, the proprioceptive and auditory memory will become permanent and will be retained years after learning each of these lessons. For example, a child swims every day and eventually becomes a good swimmer. Then after ten years with no swimming, the older child dives into the water and immediately swims with confidence. The movements of swimming are automatically felt in the memory system and are retained at the same high level skill as spoken language and listening.

SGAV: Application in Schools

To be successful, the SGAV method should be part of the preschool, kindergarten, and first grades curriculum for all children. This is the opportunity when they are able to obtain and retain the rhythm and intonation patterns of the second language. By learning the second language in each situation, young children learn to be bilingual. Through after-school clubs or particular situations in communities, a total immersion in a second language could take place. If the school system waits until middle school or high school to teach a second language, it is more difficult and the results will not be as good. If the groundwork is laid at kindergarten and first grades on the rhythm and intonation patterns, middle school and high school instruction could be used to refine the perception and reproduction of individual phonemes and prosody.

But, if by chance, people have not had the opportunity to learn a foreign language in their young age, there remains one possibility: a first training with nursery rhymes or rhythmic stimuli in space. They may not become full-fledged hearers or speakers but they can reach a certain level of fluency. A saying found in Oriental wisdom goes like this: "To learn by one's own body." It is very true for the mother tongue and the foreign languages as well.

SGAV: Application in the Private Sector

The SGAV can be used in the private sector by teaching the second language for adults in groups of up to 15 students. After the 60 hours of making the brain and the ear more sensitive to the second language, the second language SGAV can be taught through books of reading and writing. This can be independent work by the adults. However, it is critical that the first 60 to 90 hours be in the classroom with a well-trained SGAV teacher who has certification.

Summary

In summary, the SGAV method is the same Verbotonal strategy that is used for all communication problems including preschool deafness. The stages of learning and the techniques are similar. The errors that an adult of a second language makes are very similar to the errors made by a person with a hearing impairment. The second language learner is hard-of-hearing for that language because the native language interferes (i.e., the tongue [articulators] blocks the ear and the brain resists the intrusion of another language).

In addition, Americans learning Spanish will have a different pattern of errors than native French speakers learning Spanish. It is important that the teacher understand the system of errors so that they can adopt a correction procedure that is effective for that second language. This means that every American when learning Spanish will have to follow the same system. This system is different from the one that native speakers of Italian (or any other language) follow when learning Spanish.

Needless to say, such a basic training could be used for people or children suffering from speech problems, speech deficiencies, and also from speech differences. The case of dialectic or local differences is appalling in our country. We should be aware of this problem and bring an easy solution as early as possible.

References

Guberina, P. (1972). *The correlation between sensitivity of the vestibular system, and hearing and speech in Verbotonal rehabilitation* (Appendix 6, pp. 256–260). Washington, DC: Office of Vocational Rehabilitation, Department of Health, Education, and Welfare.

6

Treatment Tools and Programs

Placement

The Vestibular, Auditory, Speech, and Second Language strategies (chapters 2-6) used the treatment tools listed in Table 6–1. A reader, teacher, or parent may ask, "Where does my child begin?" Table 6–2 attempts to answer this question by identifying the following four listening performance levels: Speech Awareness, Speech Pattern Recognition, Closed-Set Recognition, and Open-Set Recognition. For example, under the Speech Awareness level, the child is not aware of speech input, especially if visual cues are reduced. His speech performance includes poor control of phonation, poor voice quality, unintelligible speech, and a possible problem in body coordination (see Table 6–2).

The appropriate treatment tools would be vestibular exercises with phonation, whole body movements, vibrotactile speech input, and rhythm and intonation stimulation. The clinician would target vowels in the low- to mid-frequency zones, for example, /u,o,a/, and consonants, for example, /m,b,p/. The vestibular exercises with phonation would be done in a straight line following the teacher's model, for example, toe-to-heel walking with /pa/pa/pa/ voicing. The whole body movements in a half-circle would highlight the parameters, duration and tension. The vibrotactile speech input through a wrist-vibrator would allow the child to feel and become aware of speech. This vocal stimulation with movement helps the child develop the listening skills for speech pattern recognition (see Table 6–2).

Table 6-1. Verbotonal Treatment Tools Based on Treatment Strategies

---

I. General
  A. Rhythm and intonation speech patterns as the foundation of both listening and speaking skills

II. Vestibular
  A. Body movements: Parameter and phoneme-based
  B. Vestibular exercises: Vocalizing while moving to develop gross and fine motor skills

III. Auditory
  A. Low to high frequency (tonality) zones: vowels, consonants, words, and sentences
  B. Verbotonal training unit: Headsets, acoustic filters, and vibrotactile speech input
  C. Distance and adverse listening practice: Unaided, hearing aid(s), or cochlear implant

IV. Speech
  A. Stimulus-response paradigm with error analysis and indirect correction
  B. Speech modification: Parameter and phoneme-based
  C. Speech rhymes: Expand the preword and word level memory patterns
  D. Situational dialogue: First, observing; and later, interaction and role-playing

---

Once the child has speech pattern recognition with reduced visual cues and has some vowel and consonant productions, he understands speech in a closed-set test format, for example, speech discrimination between four two-syllable words: "mama, baby, puppy, and daddy." As his mean utterance length increases, he can produce and understand short phrases.

For open-set speech recognition, the child should have word productions with natural coarticulation patterns and higher speech intelligibility (see Table 6–2). The acoustic filter of the Verbotonal Auditory Training Unit is used to improve his listening skills and specifically his perception of high-tonality words and sentences. Situational dialogue has the child role-playing one or more parts in a story, for example, mommy, baby, and daddy in the speech dialogue. Distance practice with his hearing aid or cochlear implant and a contralateral hearing aid also facilitates better speech recognition in noise, for example, good open-set listening performance at 15 feet, with reduced visual cues. When noise and reverberation are gradually added to the condition, he maintains the same good open-set scores.

Table 6–2. Sequence of the Verbotonal Treatment Tools based on the Child's Current Listening Performance

Current Child's Performance	Verbotonal Treatment Tools
Speech Awareness • Poor control of phonation • Unintelligible speech	Verbotonal Treatment Tools Vestibular exercises with phonation Whole body movements: duration/pause Vibrotactile speech input Low tonality sounds
Speech Pattern Recognition • Some vowel production • Poor speech intelligibility	Parameter-based body movements Speech rhyme: Preword Low and mid tonality sounds and words Speech modification: Parameter-based
Closed-Set Speech Recognition • Some consonant production, • Moderate speech intelligibility	Phoneme-based body movements Speech input with filters Mid- to high-tonality words and sentences Speech rhymes: Word Situational dialogue: Peer interaction
Open-Set Speech Recognition • Word production, coarticulation • Higher speech intelligibility	Acoustic filters with headset High-tonality words and sentences Adverse/distance listening practice Error analysis-indirect correction Situational dialogue: Role-playing

As before, the child will be referred to as "he," and the Verbotonal clinician as "she." The mother will be considered the primary caregiver, but is used exclusively only for simplicity of terms.

Treatment for Infants and Toddlers

Introduction

For infants and toddlers, the Verbotonal Approach follows the principles and guidelines of early hearing detection and intervention programs designed by ASHA Joint Committee Position on Infant Hearing. The Joint Committee stressed early intervention. The committee goals include: completing early hearing detection procedures and appropriate intervention, maximizing linguistic and communicative competency and literacy, evaluation of children before three months of age, initiating intervention before six months of age, and establishing ongoing evaluation during the child's first three years.

The early Verbotonal Approach follows the committee's guidelines of: developmental timing, direct learning, breadth and flexibility, and recognition of individual differences and environmental components. The program is family-centered, includes participants from combined disciplines, addresses cultural components, and uses informed parent choices.

Early Hearing Detection

The early hearing detection program should be a Medical-Education Model, whereby the child's pediatrician and otolaryngologist are in partnership with the parents and a certified audiologist. The audiologist is responsible for early identification and coordinating an effective aural habilitation program. The physicians provide medical clearance so the audiologist can work effectively.

Because more than 30% of children with hearing loss have additional disabilities, the child's diagnosis must be comprehensive. Some of these disabilities may be from a vestibular disorder. Guberina (1972) and Asp and Guberina (1981) reported a positive correlation between the level of hearing loss and a vestibular disorder. In other words, as the level (severity) of hearing loss increases, the incidence of a vestibular disorder increases. The vestibular disorder can also manifest in infants with normal pure-tone thresholds (i.e., children with severe expressive language deficits or an auditory processing disorder). A vestibular evaluation should be administered to these children because the test results will assist the Verbotonal clinician in planning an effective treatment program. For example, vestibular exercises are included in the habilitative program.

Other types of disabilities or medical problems that may result in hearing loss include the use of toxic drugs, a genetic component, a middle ear infection (otitis media), and so forth. A middle ear infection will create a conductive hearing loss of 30 dB HTL or greater. In addition to the tests, skilled medical care is also needed throughout the treatment program.

Verbotonal Family-Centered, Clinician-Directed Program

The Grieving Process

When the parent(s) or caregivers are first informed about their child's hearing loss, they go through very stressful stages of denial, guilt, grief, and so forth. For the first time, they realize their child is not perfect, and that the hearing loss is out of their control. Most parents feel helpless and have difficulty accepting their child's disability. The dream of a perfect baby is destroyed. Even though the mother is usually the primary caregiver, the father and siblings need to be involved in a family-centered program. All family members need to be educated and given guidance in dealing with the stages of guilt. Educating the family is an essential part of an effective program.

Counseling

The Verbotonal clinician, along with other certified professionals, provides regular educational counseling for all involved family members. The clinician helps the parents understand and talk through their feelings and emotions throughout the grieving process. The family counseling is individual and/or in small groups. The family members need to be reassured that they are not alone, so opportunities to interact with other families dealing with similar situations is often helpful. Grandparents and siblings can play an important role and should be included in the counseling sessions. The caregivers will need emotional support both from professionals and their loved ones. E-mail is used to communicate with the family to provide information between clinical visits. The parents are encouraged to use the Internet for more information.

Family Decisions

After being informed through counseling, the parents should investigate the different intervention options and programs available to their child. They should evaluate how the children in various programs are progressing and also consider children at all age-levels. The informed parents will make an informed decision on the mode of communication and the program that will best fit the needs of their child.

　　If the parents select the Verbotonal Approach, they need to understand that their child's spoken language will develop slowly at first. Once a rhythm and intonation foundation is established, the child's spoken language will improve at a faster pace.

The Mommy-Baby Method

For infants, the Verbotonal Approach follows the techniques used naturally by most dedicated mothers. These techniques are referred to as "motherese" or the "Mommy-Baby Method" (Guberina, 1972). The maternal instincts of an affectionate mother involves her holding the infant closely while singing or talking in a motherese language. Motherese involves speaking directly to the infant and is characterized by simplicity, consistency, redundancy, and exaggerated rhythm and intonation patterns. The vocal patterns, while holding the infant closely, build a strong emotional bond between the infant and the parent and facilitate the child's acquisition of an auditory-based spoken language. For an infant with a hearing impairment, the close body contact between the mother and her infant allows the infant to feel the mother's vocal patterns through the resonance within the mother's upper body. This is a basic form of vibrotactile speech input, which is especially important when the infant does not hear the mother's vocal patterns in the beginning.

Infant Speech Input

All infants have the curiosity to explore their environment by feeling, tasting, smelling, seeing, and hearing everything around them. The exploring begins in a secure environment where the infant feels his mother's vocal rhythms, while she holds him closely (vibrotactile speech input). The infant's curiosity is stimulated so he develops the desire to communicate with his mother and others around him. While being held close to his mother's body, the infant feels the emotional bond with his mother. This emotional bond then provides the foundation for the infant exploring his environment in other situations. While being held close, he learns to use his emotional vocalizations to interact with his mother. The interaction that occurs when he vocalizes teaches him that he can manipulate his environment to fulfill his needs.

The emotional link that is established between an infant and his mother provides a basis for his preword dialogue. It is established through vibrotactile speech input. The technical term is Vibra-Body speech input, an initial stage of the communication link.

Four Stages of Vibrotactile Speech Input

The four stages of the Verbotonal vibrotactile speech input are: (1) Vibra-Body, (2) Vibra-Crib, (3) Vibra-Board, and (4) Vibra-Wrist speech stimulation.

Vibra-Body Stimulation

As described above, the mother holds her infant closely in her arms while she sings or talks to him in her motherese language. The infant feels his mother's speech vibrations throughout his body. This is an example of a Verbotonal optimal learning condition. To maximize the stimulation, the mother uses a wide range of emotions in her speech patterns to help the infant feel her speech rhythm. These emotions result in wide changes in intonation speech patterns. This close physical bond between the infant and his mother is a natural instinct for both of them. It occurs during breast or formula feeding, bath time, social time, and so forth. It is called Vibra-Body stimulation; it is natural and effective for the infant because it is a secure environment for him to use preword vocalizations. These experiences intensify the infant's desire to use speech to communicate and interact with others. Because it is not possible for the mother to always hold her infant, other methods of vibrotactile speech input are needed.

Vibra-Crib Stimulation

While the infant is lying or sitting on the crib board, the mother uses the Verbotonal strategy with a microphone from the Verbotonal Auditory Training Unit to enhance her motherese spoken language input. The microphone picks up her vocal patterns and amplifies them through a vibrotactile speech vibrator that is attached to the bottom of the crib board. The crib mattress is removed so that the infant can feel the vibration directly. The entire crib board vibrates, while the infant is lying or sitting on it. This is considered a Verbotonal optimal learning condition because most of the infant's body is in contact with the vibrating crib board. The mother's speech input is the same as if she held her infant close to her body. The infant becomes sensitized to the body stimulation, so the Vibra-Crib stimulation is an alternative secure learning situation in which the infant feels his mother's vocal patterns. The Vibra-Crib stimulation begins in the clinic program, where the Verbotonal clinician demonstrates to the mother how to hold the microphone to enhance her vocal patterns. As the infant comfortably sits or lies on the crib floor, the parent follows the clinician's demonstration by speaking into the microphone and gently vibrating the crib board. The infant learns to expect and wait for the pleasant feelings of his mother's vocal patterns. With a long microphone cord, the mother can stand at a conversational distance of 3 feet, or increase her distance to 20 feet. At both distances, the infant learns to use vocalizations to communicate, because both distances provide him the same secure vocal patterns of his mother.

Vibra-Board Stimulation

For the next stage, the Vibra-Board is used for older infants and toddlers. The Vibra-Board is the same as the crib stimulation, except the board is a small wood table with short legs. The table has three vibrators attached to the bottom of it. As before, the microphone picks up the mother's vocal patterns and passes them through the Verbotonal Auditory Training Unit, where they are amplified through the attached speech vibrator. The board and the training unit are portable so it can be used in the clinic or in the mother's home. Usually, the mother's training begins on the clinic's board and continues later on a board in her home.

The board is sturdy and can handle all sizes of children. Initially, the toddler will probably want his shoes on, but he will gradually become comfortable standing, while wearing his socks. As before, this maximizes the vibrations of the mother's vocal patterns and creates an optimal learning condition.

While on the board, the Verbotonal clinician introduces the speech vibrator by placing it under a small toy. When the clinician, parent, or child vocalizes, the toy jumps off the speech vibrator. This arouses the infant or toddler's curiosity, so he will grab and hold the speech vibrator. The vibration through the board is then turned off so the child only feels the vocal patterns through the speech vibrator in his hand.

Vibra-Wrist Stimulation

Once the infant or toddler regularly holds the speech vibrator in his hand, the speech vibrator is strapped comfortably to his wrist like a wristwatch. Whenever possible, a second speech vibrator is attached to the child's leg. He feels the speech pattern through both his wrist and leg. At this point, the toddler can sit, stand, or walk while receiving his mother's vocal speech input through the speech vibrators. The child is now completely separate from the mother, but he continues to feel the security of her vocal speech input.

The four vibrotactile speech stages described above can be used in combination with each other. For example, the mother holding the infant closely with her motherese speech input, usually proceeds and follows the other conditions. This allows the infant to be secure when a condition is modified.

These stages are important for helping the infant or toddler receive proprioceptive feedback by feeling the speech patterns. They also help him expand his proprioceptive memory and develop good vocal quality. Good voice quality is essential for developing good speech intelligibility.

On a separate point, some educators have reported that some children are tactile-defensive. This defensive posture can range from not permitting vibrotactile input to absolutely no touching by the others. It is true that some infants are cautious in the beginning, but if they are approached slowly in a secure manner, they will make the transition to being held by the mother and accepting vibrotactile speech input. The writer of this book has never encountered a child that has not eventually made this transition successfully. This of course does not include children diagnosed with severe autism.

Headsets for Auditory Stimulation

Once the vibrotactile speech input has been established with the infant or toddler, a binaural headset is used. Similar to the speech vibrator, the binaural headsets provide amplified speech input for the child. Feeling the vocal patterns first helps the child learn to hear the same vocal patterns through the binaural headset, even though he may have a severe-to-profound hearing loss. The condition of simultaneously feeling and hearing the speech input is a Verbotonal optimal learning condition. It is especially important that speech input be introduced through the binaural headset before binaural hearing aids or a monaural cochlear implant. This pre-amplification training has an extended low-frequency amplification that helps develop the child's low-frequency speech perception important for rhythm and intonation patterns. This helps the child make a smooth transition to a new binaural or monaural amplification system. Development of rhythm and intonation perception enhances his adjustment to these systems. He now is able to hear the rhythm and intonation patterns, which serve as the foundation for his perception of individual phonemes within spoken phrases.

Verbotonal Infant-Toddler Stimulation

The Power of an Imitation Strategy

Young children have a strong desire to imitate the behavior patterns of adults, especially their parents. The Verbotonal Strategy uses this desire by having the infant-toddler imitate all of the speech input provided by the clinician and the parent. For example, the clinician provides a model of a many-to-one speech rhythm, for example, /ma ma ma ma (pause) maaa/. The infant or toddler will respond with a similar or slightly different speech pattern. The Verbotonal clinician analyzes the young child's response using the seven speech parameters. Then, she modifies her next speech model to facilitate a better response from the child. Later, when the child is in the same situation, he will respond to the clinician's speech model rather than just imitate.

For example, a model of "Where's Mama?" would be answered with "There's Mama." The young child learns to switch from imitation to an answer type of response. This is part of developing normal conversational skills.

Body Movements with Speech Parameters

The Verbotonal clinician begins by moving the infant's legs or arms in rhythm with her speech model. For example, she moves the infant's legs or arms quickly for the "many-to-one" rhythm pattern, then stops the leg or arm movements, then follows with one slow movement for the one-syllable response. The Verbotonal clinician uses the seven speech parameters to guide her selection of speech models to stimulate the child. For example, she initially emphasizes different speech durations, contrasting fast and slow syllable patterns. Later, she emphasizes the intonation change with emotions to improve the young child's range of intonation patterns. The body movement helps the young child feel simultaneous proprioceptive feedback from the co-occurring body and speech movements. This enhances the young child's development of proprioceptive memory patterns. These patterns are directly related to the child's development of auditory-based memory patterns.

The body movement also facilitates the infant-toddler's development of "turn-taking." The pause in movement and the speech model helps the young child learn the appropriate timing of a response. The pause sets up the response pattern for the young child. This is turn-taking, that is, the Verbotonal clinician provides the speech model and the young child responds.

Because the classical research literature reports that some infants cease vocalizing at about nine months of age, the Verbotonal clinician provides a framework for the infant to receive speech feedback. This feedback allows the infant to continue vocalizing. The feedback is through the body movements, the speech model, the vibrator, and the binaural headsets of the Verbotonal Auditory Training Unit. Feedback patterns and memory are the key to the young child's development of normal rhythm, intonation, and voice quality.

Normal Voice Quality

The Verbotonal clinician uses the parameter of tension to vary the young child's use of muscular tension in his response. These tension variations teach the child to move his speech articulators to the extreme positions. For example, he will learn to move from a low vowel, /a/, to a high vowel, /i/. The vowel /i/ is different because it is a high-tonality vowel, and it requires the child to reach high in his oral cavity to produce it correctly. Also, the change in muscular tension helps the child transition from a low, relaxed intonation to a high, tense intonation pattern. These wide and rapid changes in tension are felt through the speech vibrations. This feedback helps the infant-toddler to develop normal voice quality, which is needed for normal speech intelligibility and for the child to be accepted by all listeners as having normal speech patterns.

Meaningful Speech Stimulations

The infant-toddler will only continue to vocalize in turn-taking if the Verbotonal clinician's stimulation is meaningful and presented in a secure environment. This is why the speech model is presented with some pleasant and soft toys that are meaningful to the child. The toys accompany the speech model, for example, the toy baby moves as the clinician does a many-to-one speech rhythm. The toy needs to be changed periodically to maintain a high level of interest, and it needs to fit the mode of the speech model.

The speech rhythm patterns need to be repeated many times so the young child feels secure and has sufficient time to internalize the speech rhythm. The next section describes how situational teaching helps the young child develop speech dialogue that is meaningful to him.

Situational Teaching: The Five Stages

Introduction

The goal of situational teaching is to provide both real and imaginary conversational speech dialogue that is interesting to a curious child or group of children. These situations are introduced within the visual context of a short story that typifies everyday spoken dialogue. These situations become meaningful to the young child. The situations have characters that are real, for example, mommy, daddy, baby, puppy, and so forth. The characters can be represented by Fisher-Price toy characters, with each toy clearly identified as a specific character. In the beginning, the clinician uses only one vowel with a wide emotional range, or short syllables in a prespeech mode. Later, she adds short words, e.g. mommy, daddy, baby, and so forth.

The clinician draws the infant or toddler into the speech dialogue of the short story. The speech dialogue begins with simple spoken language, for example, "Hi Mommy," and gradually advances to a more complex spoken language, for example, "Mommy went to the store." The clinician draws the young child into the situational story by using common spoken language of the child's home environment. Slowly, the young child begins to interact, and most importantly, remembers the spoken dialogue of the characters.

The clinician uses an optimal learning condition by providing vibrotactile speech input from the speech vibrator on a vibratory board and/or on the child's wrist. The young child feels the rhythm and intonation patterns of the clinician as well as his verbal response to the situations. As soon as possible, the binaural headset is added to the speech vibrator so the child can both feel and hear the speech patterns of all the characters.

The five stages of situational teaching are a gradual progression from simple speech dialogues to more complex spoken interactions. The Verbotonal clinician is skilled in using simple, closed spoken phrases that are appropriate for the child's developmental age, for example, "Where's Mommy?" or "Hi Puppy." For a four-year-old with a developmental age of two years, the clinician uses speech that is appropriate for the two-year level.

Stage 1: Clinician-Directed

The Verbotonal clinician (as an actress) uses her spontaneous emotions to portray a meaningful short story, for example, "Hi Mommy, Where's Daddy, Hi Puppy, Let's walk, Walk-Walk-Walk." The toy character is moved in harmony with each of the clinician's spoken utterances in an action fitting for the short story. The clinician uses a variety of spoken emotions to make the story meaningful, for example., surprise, happy, and so on. The spoken emotions are used with the appropriate body language to make the emotions meaningful.

In Stage 1 the infant or toddler watches closely and develops an interest in what the toy characters are doing and saying. Although this stage is clinician- (or mommy-) directed, the goal is to entice the young child to participate in the spoken dialogue. Once the child begins to participate, Stage 2 begins.

Stage 2: Child Participates

The clinician encourages the young child to be one of the characters in the story. The clinician always accepts how the young child plays the toy character and interacts with the other toy character(s). For example, he imitates the puppy walking or running with /ba ba ba baaa/. The clinician moves the child's hand while he holds the toy puppy and moves it with the same speech rhythm that the child is vocalizing. The child receives both tactile and proprioceptive feedback from his simultaneous arm movement and his spoken syllables. This enhances his proprioceptive memory for simultaneous vocalization patterns.

Stage 3: Child Assumes More Responsibility

The clinician raises her expectations of the young child and uses her modifications to improve the child's spoken responses. At the beginning, the young child only imitates what the clinician says. Later, the young child will add his or her own vocalizations, for example, a surprise reaction of "Uh oh" when the puppy falls. The short stories become more complex during Stage 3, and the child takes more responsibility in the speech dialogue. For example, the child may play two or three characters in the same story.

Stage 4: Child Becomes More Creative

The young child begins to add new spoken language to the speech dialogue to enhance the short story. The child progresses from imitative responses to creative spoken language, adding details and personal knowledge to the interactions. The creativity shows that the young child has mastered and remembers the entire spoken language in the short story. He now wants to expand by using other phrases, for example, "The baby says /ba ba ba ba/" or "Where's the baby?" or "There's the baby."

Stage 5: Child Role-Plays the Story

The child plays one or more of the characters without props and without cues from the clinician. At this stage one or two young children can take turns by each role-playing a character in the story. The children can practice the short story situation until they have mastered all the spoken language. Then, they can perform the short story for an interested audience of other clinicians and family members.

Stage 5 can be continued with older children and with more advanced levels of speech dialogue. A high level of speech dialogue was performed in Zagreb, Croatia at the recent International Verbotonal Conference. The Verbotonal school-age children put on the opera, "Mid-Summer Night's Dream" in a formal stage performance. These children used English, French, and Croatian dialogue to demonstrate their mastery of these three spoken languages. The children had practiced their roles for months in preparation for the final performance. The final stage is unlimited in the complexity of the spoken language, length of the story, and the number of characters involved. Because the children are role-playing as actors, they have the opportunity to greatly expand their language skills.

Transition to School-Based Program

The Verbotonal infant-toddler, parent-based program uses the binaural headsets and vibrotactile speech stimulation to develop his auditory perception of rhythm and intonation speech patterns. These speech patterns connect the child's phoneme perception of individual speech sounds. In other words, the individual speech sounds are learned on top of the suprasegmental patterns.

The Verbotonal clinician develops a rapport with a school-based Verbotonal program that is state-funded and provides a free education to all children beginning at three years of age. The Verbotonal clinician educates the child's family with written information and visits to the school-based program. When the child's Individual Education Plan (IEP) is developed, the parent and all involved professionals will decide if the child should be placed in a mainstream classroom or a self-contained class with partial mainstreaming. The Verbotonal clinician helps to provide a smooth transition for the child and his family.

Treatment for School-Aged Children

Introduction

In the United States, the Verbotonal Approach began in 1964 and has continued to develop for the past 38 years at the University of Tennessee Verbotonal Research Lab. During this period, it was implemented in both a small (60,000 children) and a large (500,000 children) public school system; these are Knox County (1975 to present) and Miami-Dade County (1984 to present), respectively. Both school systems have a full-day preschool class for three-year-olds who have a delay in their aural-oral communication skills. These Verbotonal classes provide an auditory-based communication foundation for the children so that they may successfully be mainstreamed in kindergarten or elementary school levels. After the child is mainstreamed, there is follow-up treatment at all levels, including the high school students.

Knox and Miami-Dade County Schools both mainstream over 80% of their children into regular school classrooms with minimal accommodations. Most of these children graduate from high school with a regular high school diploma, and many continue their education and get college degrees. In short, the children successfully complete the regular school curriculum, which prepares them to be competitive in the academic and/or work environments.

The success of the Verbotonal Approach is based on well-trained clinicians who skillfully implement the strategy. The Verbotonal clinicians use error analysis and the treatment tools to correct each child at the appropriate developmental levels using the Verbotonal Auditory Training Unit. This unit provides an optimal listening condition for each child to maximize both their spoken language and their listening skills. The optimum learning condition is a wide-frequency response, including the extended low frequencies with a speech vibrator and binaural headsets. Some researchers have reported that children need a wider frequency bandwidth than adults. The children with hearing loss continue to use their binaural hearing aids or their monaural cochlear implant, after school. Some of these children do not need an FM wireless system, because they have well-developed listening skills. This section describes how this strategy is successfully implemented into a regular public school structure and curriculum. It also provides examples of how the Verbotonal Strategy has been effective.

School Structure

Responsibility

Public school systems are legally responsible for educating all children within their school district. Accountability of the teachers and the school is primarily judged by the children's ability to read at or above their grade level. The academic success of the children affects the appropriation of state and local funding; therefore, emphasis is placed on academics rather than social skills.

It is the school system's responsibility to provide the least restrictive environment for children with disabilities, with as much access to the regular classroom curriculum as possible. A multidisciplinary team meets with the parents of disabled children to approve an appropriate Individualized Education Plan (IEP). This plan includes the procedures, goals, and objectives for the child. When appropriate, the Verbotonal Strategy is part of the child's IEP.

Parent-Assisted

As part of the strategy, parents or caregivers are responsible for the child's attendance and are encouraged to attend school activities and participate in the Parent Teacher Association (PTA). Parents are encouraged to assume an active role in their child's education. Whenever possible, the Verbotonal Strategy includes parents in the child's educational program, for their involvement is necessary to have daily communication and follow-up practice of communication skills in the home.

Preparation for a School-Based Program

An effective Clinic Infant-Toddler Program described earlier prepares the child and parent for a smooth transition to the school-based program. This begins by having the appropriate school official involved in planning the young child's Individual Family Service Plan (IFSP). The school system, in turn, involves the Clinic Program Director as a consultant in the child's IEP. This cooperative communication between the clinic program and the school system maximizes the child's adjustment to the school-based program.

In some cases, infants and toddlers who were not enrolled in a clinic program begin a school-based program without the basic communication and behavioral skills training. In other cases, children were transferred from a clinic program that was in competition with the school program. This competition often confuses the parents because of the difference in goals of the clinic program and the state-monitored school program. When this mismatch occurs, it has a negative effect on the child's development. When this type of confusion occurs, it should be addressed and resolved in the school IEP meeting.

Regardless of the child's circumstances, the school system is responsible for selecting a multidisciplinary team (M-TEAM). The M-TEAM develops the goals and objectives for each child's Individualized Education Plan. Before the IEP meeting, each child is assessed in six major areas: (1) communication, (2) self-help, (3) prevocational, (4) pre-academics, (5) motor (fine and gross), and (6) social skills. The child's disorder must affect one or more of these skills to qualify him for a special education status. Detailed information from the infant clinic program is helpful in developing an effective IEP.

Discipline

The Verbotonal strategy follows a strong and effective discipline policy in a friendly, loving atmosphere (tough-love). The policy is easy to implement because most school systems have a zero-tolerance disciplinary policy that applies to all children, including those with communication disorders. All children need a clear view of what is expected of them and what types of behavior will and will not be tolerated. A tough-love strategy in a friendly atmosphere tends to produce the most effective results. The clinician establishes behavioral control, promotes good team spirit, and ensures that each child feels comfortable and accepted. The clinician helps the parent apply the same behavior management at home. Good classroom discipline with follow-up at home is the basis for maximizing the learning potential of each child.

Treatment Tools

Verbotonal Strategy

The Verbotonal strategy is based on teaching effective listening skills to develop good voice quality and intelligible conversational speech. Initially, the young child imitates the clinician's vocal stimulation/model using preword rhythm and intonation patterns. The child eventually progresses to words, phrases, and sentences. The clinician's vocal stimulations are always used in a meaningful context so the child's response is meaningful. Later, the child's dominant listening skills will help him self-correct his speech errors.

Treatment for Children

The following is a list of the Verbotonal treatment tools: stimulus-response paradigm, speech parameters, speech modification, vibrotactile speech input, binaural headset input, filtered speech, vestibular exercises, body movements, speech rhymes, memory span, tonality progression, tonality words, situational teaching, error analysis, didactic/incidental learning, and the transition from the Verbotonal Auditory Training Unit to the personal auditory aids of the child. These treatment tools were discussed earlier in this book. The clinician uses these tools for error analysis and speech modification to correct the child's language response and listening skills. The clinician's goal is to create the optimal learning condition for each child. There is a normal developmental progression as the child becomes competent in his listening and spoken language skills. These aural-oral skills serve as a foundation for academic success within the regular school curriculum, just as they do for children with normal hearing. This is a basic assumption of the Verbotonal strategy.

Verbotonal Auditory Training Units

Verbotonal Strategy

The auditory strategy includes the consistent use of a wide-band, extended low-frequency response. As the child experiences success, he wears the binaural headsets and the speech vibrator of the Verbotonal Auditory Training Unit throughout the school day. This success develops his auditory confidence. After school, the child uses his personal binaural hearing aid(s). Children with a monaural cochlear implant wear their implant with the speech vibrator and a monaural headset on the nonimplanted side. The consistent, daily use of a binaural, wide-band speech signal in a quiet environment is critical for developing each child's listening skills.

Most Comfortable Loudness (MCL)

The clinician uses the child's audiometric pure-tone average (e.g., 60 dB HL) and speech reception threshold (e.g., 65 dB HL) for estimating the appropriate loudness level in each earphone of the Verbotonal Auditory Training Unit. The clinician adjusts the volume control on the five-station rack in an ascending-descending order to establish the child's speech reception threshold (SRT) in each ear. The child imitates what the clinician says, for example, /ma ma/. The child's MCL level is set above his SRT. Next, a specialized sound-level-meter, with an insert microphone in each earphone, is used to measure the sound pressure level (SPL) of the teacher's speech input. The SPL of the clinician's voice has to agree with the estimated level from the Child's PTA and SRT. As the child becomes a better listener, he or she is able to set his or her own MCL and needs less amplification (SPL) to achieve the same loudness. The SPL meter is consistently used to verify the appropriate loudness level for the child. This eliminates the possibility of overamplification.

Different Hearing Levels in the Same Classroom

As described above, setting a pleasant MCL in both the child's left and right earphones is critical for developing his listening skills. For example, a child with a profound hearing loss and a child with normal pure-tone thresholds each have their own unique MCL. The Verbotonal Auditory Training Unit is adjusted in loudness to provide a pleasant level for each child. Normal-hearing children are included if they have unintelligible speech and poor listening skills. Setting individual loudness levels allows children with different disorders to be included in the same classroom. For example, the MCL is made comfortable by setting the clinician's speech input at 105 dB SPL for a child with a severe hearing impairment, and 65 dB SPL (a 40 dB difference) for a child with normal hearing. As a result, both of these children will experience a pleasant loudness of the clinician's voice.

A Wide Bandwidth

The wide bandwidth (2 to 20,000 Hz) of the Model I Verbotonal Auditory Training Unit is used to maximize the binaural speech input to stimulate the child's brain. The child is able to simultaneously feel (speech vibrator) and hear (binaural headset) the clinician's speech input. With the broad bandwidth set at the child's MCL, the low-frequency zone is stimulated and developed first. This zone is optimal for perceiving the rhythm and intonation speech patterns. In addition, a low-pass filter is added to enhance the child's feeling of the speech rhythms. The rhythms enhance the development of the child's proprioceptive and auditory memory. After some low-pass stimulation, the teacher switches back to the broadband condition and the child makes a positive learning transfer to the broadband stimulation.

Feeling the Movement and Hearing the Speech

The vibrotactile speech input of the clinician's voice helps establish and maintain an emotional bond between the clinician and each child because each child can feel her rhythm and intonation patterns. Feeling the rhythm provides the foundation for developing the child's listening skills through the binaural headsets. At an advanced level, the auditory perception becomes the dominant modality in the child's spoken language. The clinician covers her face to reduce visual clues and facilitate a response through listening.

The vibrotactile speech feedback is also important because it helps each child to feel and control his vocal patterns. This feedback is important for establishing good voice quality, which enhances the child's speech intelligibility and increases his feelings of social acceptance from his normal-hearing peers.

Spectral Change to Refine Listening Skills

The Verbotonal Auditory Training Unit (Model II) helps to refine the child's listening skills. Model II is a five-channel unit used to create the child's optimal frequency response (OFR) for correction or for general listening skills. For example, a high-pass filter of 6000 Hz is added to a low-pass filter to correct the perceptual error, for example, "tea" for "see." The high-pass filtered condition allows the child to hear the target /s/ in the word "see" clearly, while the perception of the error, /t/, is eliminated. In this example, the low speech frequencies, which carry the rhythm and intonation patterns, make the child more sensitive to the high speech frequencies. The acoustic filters are used for an individual child or in small groups with children who have similar perceptual problems. The Verbotonal Strategy is designed for each child to refine his or her listening skills with filters in both the classroom and individual treatment.

Optimal to Adverse Listening

Once the child is stable in listening skills developed for the optimum listening condition, the Verbotonal Auditory Training Unit is used to create adverse listening conditions to prepare the child for the noisy mainstream classroom environment (e.g., +5 dB S/N ratio with reverberation). For example, the unit is set for 0.8 seconds reverberation time (delay) for the clinician's voice. Initially, this creates an adverse listening condition for the child. With the clinician using error analysis and correction, the child will gradually perceive speech in both the optimal (0.0 seconds) and the adverse (0.8 seconds) reverberation conditions with the same success. This indicates that the child has expanded his optimum condition to include both the 0.0 and the 0.8 seconds reverberation time. Next, noise is added by recording many speakers at the same time at a +5 dB S/N ratio. With practice, the child will hear the clinician's speech input at this adverse condition of +5 dB S/N ratio. Finally, the earlier reverberation condition and the noise condition are added together. This listening practice in adverse conditions prepares the child for successful listening in a noisy classroom or auditorium.

Vestibular Exercises: Balance and Space Perception

As mentioned earlier, the Knox County School System uses a vestibular exercise program (SMART Curriculum, Palmer, 1999) for all their normal-hearing children in kindergarten. These vestibular exercises are used daily to develop the child's gross and fine-motor skills. This helps prepare each child for a readiness training program, and to develop his or her reading skills.

The Verbotonal Strategy also uses the SMART Curriculum with children who have communication disorders. These vestibular exercises help prepare each child for speech stimulation using body movements and speech rhymes. The body movements are combined with his vocalizations to maximize the development of his neural plasticity and his proprioceptive memory. This helps him to learn at a faster rate and to catch up with normally developing children. The SMART curriculum (Palmer, 1999) includes exercises such as crawling, creeping, tracking, brachiation (swinging one arm to the other arm), cross-pattern walking, flashlight walking, bilateral jumping jacks, and trampoline exercises. The large muscle exercises are followed by fine-muscle activities targeted sitting at a desk. These exercises are used daily for 20 minutes. The exercises precede body movements, speech rhymes, and table activities. The clinician adapts the vestibular exercises and body movements to the motoric skills of the children. These exercises continue to develop throughout the school year.

Parameters of Listening and Speech

Stimulus-Response, Analysis, and Correction

As explained earlier, the clinician analyzes the child's speech imitation (response) and uses the analyses to modify her next speech model. Her speech modification highlights one or more parameters to provide the optimum learning condition for the child. In the beginning stage, the child imitates the clinician's first and each subsequent speech model. When the child successfully imitates the model, the optimal learning condition has been achieved. The speech parameters are the tools for both analysis and correction.

The child is instructed to imitate what he hears without guessing. This helps the clinician analyze what the child perceives. Pointing and gesturing are not accepted, because they are passive forms of listening. Imitating the clinician's body movements and speech model helps the child organize his own speech patterns.

The clinician's speech stimulations begin at the preword level and advance to the word level. The seven parameters that are listed in Table 6–3 (C. Davis, personal communication, 2005) provide examples of one, two, and three-syllable rhythm patterns. The following is a brief discussion of how each parameter is used for speech input.

Speech Parameters

Rhythm. With the clinician's gentle guidance, the young child first babbles many syllables in a spontaneous manner. Then, after perceiving the clinician's speech input, he vocalizes many syllables, a pause, and one controlled syllable; for example, /ma ma ma/ (pause) /ma/.

Table 6–3. Treatment Tools: Developmental Age Levels I, II, and III*

Tools	I: 1–2* Years (Dev. Age)	II: 2–4 Years (Dev. Age)	III: 4–5 Years (Dev. Age)
1. Parameters: Analysis (1) Rhythm (2) Intonation (3) Pause (4) Time (5) Tension (6) Pitch (7) Loudness	• speech awareness • on/off • many/one (pause) • fast/slow • long/short • loud/soft • tense/less tense	• 2–6 syllables • fast/slow timing	• 7–12 syllable with pauses
2. Speech Modification	• independent stimulation through play • correct rhythm • wide range of emotions	• direct correct. rhythms • stimulate phonemes • evaluation	• direct correct phonemes • less emotion
3. Vibrotactile Input	• vibrator board/wrist vibrator	• wrist vibrator	
4. Headset Input • Filters or Wideband	• headsets • VTU1	• headsets • filters VTU I and II	• headsets • filters • VTU I and II
5. Vestibular Exercises	• crawl/spin	• balance	• fine-motor
6. Body Movements • Parameter-based • Phonome-based	• body movements • stop and start • space perception/jump/walk	• parameter correction. • phoneme correction	• phoneme correction

Tools	I: 1–2 Years (Dev. Age)	II: 2–4 Years (Dev. Age)	III: 4–5 Years (Dev. Age)
7. Speech Rhymes • syllables • words • Phrases	• ah, boo, bah, boo, boo, boo, bah • apple apple yum yum yum apple • apple I want one!	• Oh boy, I'm happy I have a tree • Wow . . . many toys maybe . . . one's for me!	• Funny little bushy tail lives in a tree • Funny little bushy tail Will you play with me?
8. Memory Span • propioceptive • auditory	• begin many-to-one • open the door	5–7 syllables	10–16 syllables
9. Tonality • vowels • consonants • words • phrases	low-tonality vowels: [u o a] (p, b, m, n, w) mama, baby, apple mama up	low and mid-tonality vowels: [o a u] (t,d,k,g, l) daddy, car, touch don't touch	Low, mid. and high vowels: [e ɪ] (s,sh,z,c,h) sunny, cheese, zipper it's a sunny day outside
10. Situational Teaching	• teacher-directed • identification	• child participates • limited expression	• children role play • child uses spontaneous phrases and imagination
11. Didactic—Incidental • didactic • incidental	• didactic—95% • incidental—95%	• didactic—80% • incidental—20%	• didactic—50% • incidental—50%
12. Training Unit: Transition • HA • CI • Noise/reverberation	• pre-HA • pre-CI	• HA with broadband • CI worn in class with headset/ vibrator	• HA responds like filters • CI worn in class

*Prepared with the assistance of L. Davis

Once he masters a one-syllable response, he has internalized a one-syllable speech rhythm. Usually, the child can walk the same basic rhythm. The development of his vocal rhythms parallels the development of his motoric skills of his body.

As the child advances, he is able to produce a two-syllable pattern. This involves three possible duration patterns: a trochaic pattern (long-short pattern), a spondee pattern (long-long pattern), and an iambic pattern (short-long pattern). Most children go from one controlled syllable pattern to the trochaic pattern (e.g., "baby, mommy, daddy, etc."). Once these rhythmic patterns are internalized in the child's proprioceptive and auditory memory, his speech becomes more intelligible.

Intonation. The clinician begins by establishing a pleasant vocal pitch in the child's spoken productions. If the child demonstrates high or low body tension, his vocal pitch will also be too high or too low. The degree of muscular body tension corresponds to the degree of vocal tension, which is perceived as vocal pitch. While the child imitates the clinician's body movements with changing degrees of body tension, he simultaneously feels his intonation changing and experiences a pleasant vocal pitch. To help the child, the clinician's vocal patterns are paired with vibrotactile speech input on the child's wrist so that the child can feel the different types of affectivity in her voice.

The clinician uses intonation patterns that have a wide emotional range and are meaningful to the child. For example, giving a look of disgust and pointing while saying the vowel /u/ implies that something is undesirable and needs to be avoided. This is meaningful in the child's preword spoken language. The clinician changes her body language and presents it in a meaningful context so that the message is conveyed clearly. Body language in a practical situation helps the child internalize the pragmatics of his preword language patterns.

Tension. The clinician expresses tension changes by increasing and decreasing muscle tension in her body movements and her vocal patterns. These tension changes help the child to experience proprioceptive feedback for his utterances. For example, the clinician increases her body's muscle tension contractions in a wide-sweeping, upward arm movement as she vocalizes an upward intonation pattern in a vowel, for example, /a/. The child's simultaneous imitation of the movement helps him feel the change in intonation.

Each phoneme has a typical level of muscle tension; for example, the vowel /i/ has greater tension than the vowel /a/. Also, the consonant /p/ has more muscle tension than the consonant /m/. Even though each phoneme in isolation has a typical tension for categorical perception, the tension is increased or decreased in coarticulation to emphasize the quality of each phoneme. For example, with the least tense vowel, /a/, the tension can be increased or decreased with certain limits and only the quality changes. If the tension change is too great, a different vowel will be categorically perceived. For consonants, too much tension forces the child to categorically perceive tense /b/ for a less tense target /m/. Conversely, if the muscle tension is decreased for the target, /m/, the child perceives the less tense /m/. The tension parameter is an effective treatment tool for both categorical phoneme perception and suprasegmental perception.

Pause. The clinician uses pause as an effective treatment tool for speech rhythms. For example, in the basic speech rhythm, "many-to-one," there is a pause with tension before the one controlled syllable. Walking and pausing while phonating is a basic technique for the child to use when producing the "many-to-one" speech rhythm. The child walks and phonates with the same rhythm. The simultaneous phonation and moving enhance the child's proprioceptive memory.

Pitch. The clinician begins by vocalizing the low-tonality phonemes and syllables to develop the child's perceptions within the low-frequency zone, for example, /u,a,b,m/. Once the low-zone is established, the clinician moves to the mid-tonality zone, for example, /t,d,k,g/, and so forth. The tonality of the phonemes and syllables follows the phonemic developmental order of normal-hearing children. The tonality zones are based on the child's auditory perceptions and are used as an effective tool for teaching the child the necessary skills for intelligible speech and listening skills.

Loudness. The clinician changes the loudness of her vocalizations and the child perceives them as very loud to very soft. Then, the child imitates the clinician's loudness and uses body movement variations to vary his own loudness. These changes help the child develop proprioceptive feedback for loudness control. Also, by teaching him to produce a pleasant vocal loudness in a variety of situations, the clinician is teaching him to use self-control and to be consistent.

Duration and Tempo. In harmony with her body movements, the clinician changes her speech tempo from slow (2 syllables/second) to normal (5 syllables/second) to fast (8 syllables/second). The child imitates her movements and her vocalizations, using the same speech tempo. This helps the child to vary his speech tempo. In the beginning the clinician uses a slow tempo. It is an optimal condition, because the child needs more time to perceive and produce the speech patterns. Later, a quicker vocal tempo with body movements is used to expand the child's capacity for perceiving the quickened tempo. In both examples the optimal learning condition is used; the second condition is also optimal because the child expands his ability to process eight syllables/second.

Verbotonal Treatment Tools: Three Developmental Age Levels

Verbotonal Strategy

The clinician uses the treatment tools in Table 6–3 to stimulate and correct the child's spoken language, which is based on his or her listening skills. In short, the clinician uses suprasegmental and segmental speech patterns to develop functional listening skills for speech. Table 6–3 is divided into three developmental age levels: Level One: 1 to 2 years, Level Two: 2 to 4 years, and Level Three: 4 to 5 years. For example, a three-year-old deaf child may have a one-year developmental speech age. With this two-year delay, this child must learn at a fast rate to catch up with his normal developing peers. In other words, a learning rate of 1.5 years/year is needed for a child with a communication disorder to "catch-up."

The speech parameters, voice modification, and the Verbotonal Auditory Training Unit were discussed earlier; now body movements, vestibular exercises, speech rhymes, tonality, and situational teaching are discussed.

Verbotonal Vestibular Exercises and Body Movements

The vestibular exercises develop the child's balance, coordination, and "perception in space." They are used in harmony with vocalizations. Body movements are also used with vocalizations to develop the child's proprioceptive and auditory feedback for processing spoken language.

The body movements begin with parameter-based stimulation and later phoneme-based stimulation. Initially, indirect stimulation is used so the child feels free to express himself without being directly corrected. The child is unaware of the indirect stimulation strategy; he simply enjoys the movements while he vocalizes. At the second and third levels, the clinician uses direct correction, because the child's voice quality, rhythm, and intonation patterns have been internalized and stabilized. He now sounds like a normal hearing preschooler. In short, direct correction is only used with a socially secure child with stable rhythm and intonation patterns.

Speech Rhymes

The purpose of speech rhymes is to increase the child's proprioceptive and auditory memory (Table 6–3). The body movements are used to highlight the rhythm and reinforce the child's memory. Level One begins by teaching a seven-syllable preword rhyme, for example, "a boo, bah boo, boo, boo, bah." At the later stage, the clinician uses an eight-word speech rhyme: "apple, apple, yum yum yum, I want some." In short, both of these rhymes are taught one line at a time until the child can remember more than one line. Some of the speech rhymes have a concentration of one phoneme. For example, "Um-um, uma-um, mu mee, mommy" concentrates on the /m/ phoneme. This facilitates mastery of the /m/ sound in a meaningful rhythm with a series of coarticulations.

The child's memory span begins with the many-to-one syllable rhythm, and later develops to a two and three-syllable rhythm. By Level Two, the memory span is 6 to 10 syllables; and by Level Three, it is 10 to 16 syllables. A Level Three memory span is needed for the child to participate in a normal speech dialogue with a peer or caring adult.

Phonemes Based in Tonality Zones

As mentioned earlier, the clinician begins with low-tonality syllables, /pa, ba, ma, mu, bu, mu/, and advances to low tonality words, "mama, baby, apple, up, bus, big," and so forth. Later, she uses mid-tonality syllables, /ta, da, ka, ga/, and advances to "daddy, car, touch," and so forth. At an advanced stage, she uses the high-tonality syllables, /si, shi, ti, zi/, and advances to words such as "sunny, cheese, seat, zipper," and so forth. These tonality zones give the clinician direction for planning lessons.

Situational Teaching: Pragmatic Skills

There are five stages of situational teaching discussed earlier; clinician-directs, child participates, child assumes more responsibility, child becomes creative, and child role-plays the story. These real and imaginary situations allow the child to experience turn-taking, topic maintenance, active questioning, and using the rules of spoken interactions. These situations provide the context for the child to develop the necessary pragmatic skills of a speech dialogue.

Curriculum

Verbotonal Strategy

The strategy of the preschool curriculum is to provide the child with appropriate spoken language skills. Table 6–4 (Davis & Asp, 2005) provides some examples of the three developmental levels of the "I Like School" curriculum.

Curriculum: I Like School

A thorough understanding of language concepts is necessary for the child to effectively use spoken language and to be successful with different academic subjects. In Level One, concepts are contrasted, such as "up-down, in-out, big-little, go-stop," whereas negative concepts "no" and "not" are simply introduced in an appropriate context. At Level Two the concepts include "on-off, fast-slow, wet- (not wet) dry, dirty- (not dirty) clean," and so forth. "Not wet" is used before "dry" and "not dirty" is used before "clean." At Level Three the concepts include "many-few, front-back, forward-backward, far-near," and so forth.

Table 6–4 includes examples for words, situations, art, literature, and preacademics. These examples are useful in blending spoken language with academics. It prepares the child for academic skills of reading, writing, and spelling.

Typical School Day

The treatment tools and curriculum are implemented daily in a school day (e.g. 8:00 AM to 2:30 PM). Table 6–5 provides an example of a typical school day. It is an intensive, playful learning situation for all of the children.

Group and Individual Treatment

The Verbotonal Strategy includes both group and individual treatment. In a school-based treatment program, the group (or small classroom) treatment serves as the basis for the program. It follows the format of all school systems and combines children in small or large classes, as needed. The first part of this chapter pertains to classroom treatment; however, all children need individual treatment. Individual treatment incorporates the same strategies, only they are applied to each child's individual needs that cannot be targeted during classroom treatment.

Table 6–4. I Like School Curriculum: Developmental Age Levels

	Level I: 0–2 Years	Level II: 2–4 Years	Level III: 4–5 Years
Vowels/phonemes words	Early developing sounds M—mama, me, I'm more B—bus, boy, big, bye P—up, open, puppy W—wake, wow, one	Level 1 sounds and T—two, put, out, time D—don't, bed, do K—come, can cake G—go, gone, get	Level 1, 2 sounds and S—bus, pants, cereal Z—buzz, zip, zoom SH—shhh, shoe, show CH—lunch, ouch
Situations	Bye mama, I'm on the bus Wake up, not me, mama boy on the bus, open the door, Where's? Who's?	get up—get on the bus get out of bed, put on my . . . I can___. Time to ___ I want, I have, is verbing	shh, I'm sleeping Ouch, I bumped my head zoom . . . go fast, not slow Can I have, Do you have
Concepts	up/down go/stop big/little not in/out	on/off fast/slow wet/not wet/dry dirty/not dirty/clean	many/few far/near close front/back forward/backward
Art	tissue paper/yellow bus	cut/paste bus parts	follow oral directions—put bus together—cut parts
Literature Activity	wheels on the bus large bus—put people on as large group	wheels on the bus individual folder game follow along—fill in missing words	wheels on the bus sing song—act out
Situational Teaching	teacher directed wake-up—sequence story	teacher/student interaction teacher directs—student interaction	student-directed spontaneous language
Pre/Academic	match colors-crayons string macaroni wheels of various colors	receptively identify colors follow teacher pattern of specific colors	expressively name colors follow teacher pattern of specific colors/shapes

Table 6–5. Daily Routine for a Full Day Program*

Time	Activity
8:00–8:30	Arrive/bathroom/Daily routine Social language, Vocabulary, Questions/Answers Hearing Aid Check, Prevocational skills—caring for personal belongings.
8:30–9:00	Vestibular exercises—spinning, crawling w/natural vocalizations Breakfast Social language, Vocabulary, Questions/Answers Targeted phrases, vocabulary, rhythm patterns Example: I want ___ and ___ and___.
9:00–10:45	Large Group-Training Unit (headsets and vibrators) Sound stimulation Stimulus/Response through Situational Teaching Suprasegmentals: (e.g.) Level 1: Imitation Level 2: Imitation/communicative intent Level 3: natural voice quality Parameters—rhythm, intonation, duration, intensity, pitch, pause, tension Segmentals: (e.g.) Level 1: p, b, m, n, w Level 2: all above and k, g, t, d, l Level 3: all above and s, sh, ch, z, j Targeted unit vocabulary Targeted unit phrases Targeted concepts: (e.g.) Level 1: up/down, big/little Level 2: tall/short, over/under Level 3: forward/backward, near/far Targeted rhythm patterns Teacher-directed role-play Literature-based activities—speech rhythms, stories
10:45–11:15	Art/Morning Closure Activity Something for the child to take home Fine-motor activities—cut/paste, paint Reinforces morning activities
11:15–11:30	Bathroom walk down hall in line quiet/loud gross motor/vestibular exercises—crosswalk, walk on line, Walk backward, etc.

160

Time	Activity
11:30–12:15	Lunch—family-style with teacher and teaching assistant listen for carryover—Incidental Learning targeted phrases: I want . . . I don't want . . . I like . . . I'm done, That's good, etc.
12:15–1:00	"Free play" inside or outside—listen for carryover—Incidental Learning teacher-directed activities for some children watch for parallel play listen for social interactions—initiation of activity social games—solve problems
1:00–1:30	Afternoon large group activity (Training Unit) Supplemental activities traditional games match games with unit vocabulary preacademic unit act. (colors, numbers, shapes) role play (e.g., act out "is verbing"—children guess) literature-based activities that are theme related (e.g., November—Home and Family—my version of 3 Bears)
1:30–2:00	Snack listen for carryover-related "snack" items (color, vocab.) targeted vocabulary, phrases social language—e.g., 1 child passes thing out "do you want juice?"
2:00–2:30	Small Group/Individual Therapy/Rest Time Daily small group/individual—target specific problems Training Unit Preimplant evaluations Audiologic evaluations Earmolds, repairs, etc.
2:50	Dismissal
3:00	Planning Time

*Prepared with the assistance of L. Davis.

The Verbotonal Auditory Training Unit, Model II, has five channels and filters and is used to provide optimal frequency response (OFR), which includes the optimal octave for specific phoneme correction. The highest performance outcomes occur when children receive both group and individual treatment. Individual treatment helps the child deal with his own difficulties.

Mainstreaming

Verbotonal Strategy

The goal of the Verbotonal Approach is to develop normal spoken language and listening skills so that each child can be mainstreamed into a regular classroom in his home school with minimum accommodation.

Verbotonal Auditory Training Unit: Transition to Binaural Hearing Aids

Children with a hearing impairment make the positive learning transfer from the training unit to their hearing aids or cochlear implants. Listening and speaking skills, with the necessary corrections, are a major focus of the entire school day. The clinician rewards the children for good listening and good speech. Each child internalizes these skills so that they become a part of their daily behavior. Listening is a "way of life" for all these children. In fact, they often become better listeners than children with normal hearing.

The speech stimulation through the binaural headset provides effective binaural listening through both the poorer and the better ear. Effective binaural listening is necessary for high-performance listening and localization in the reverberation and noise of a mainstream classroom. Most children wear binaural hearing aids, which make effective binaural listening a realistic goal.

Binaural Headsets to a Monaural Cochlear Implant

The binaural headset training also provides effective binaural pre-implant treatment by preparing the child's brain for the perception of speech rhythm and intonation patterns in both ears. This speech pattern perception provides a foundation for the child's successful transition to the direct electrical stimulation from his cochlear implant. The vibrotactile speech input is used with the cochlear implant to enhance the transition and to develop effective vocal control and speech for each child. A monaural earphone is placed in the contralateral ear to help these children maintain their effective binaural listening. The poorer ear is developed along with the ear that has the cochlear implant. The goal is to fit a hearing aid on the contralateral ear. This makes the child an effective binaural listener in noisy and reverberant classrooms. He can listen through a cochlear implant and a hearing aid simultaneously.

Mainstreaming Stages

Children with severe and profound hearing losses begin partial mainstreaming in a kindergarten class when they have completed developmental ages four-to-five years (Table 6–3). This partial mainstreaming prepares them for full mainstreaming into an elementary school. Whenever possible, full mainstreaming is implemented in the child's home school. Other children with moderate hearing loss, or with normal hearing, who start with unintelligible speech reach the four- to five-year developmental ages within one to two school years of intensive treatment (1,000+ hours per year). These children can be fully mainstreamed by kindergarten or first grade and can go directly to their home school program. In other words, the place and level of mainstreaming is based on each child's developmental age, which is part of the IEP.

Other forms of mainstreaming are inclusion and integration. Inclusion involves the special education teacher sitting in the classroom with the child to help assist him in successfully completing the classroom curriculum. With integration, the child has special education goals and the IEP has been modified to fit the child's potential achievements. Some children who are not completely successful in oral skills may need an oral or manual interpreter in the classroom.

Wireless Systems

With an effective Verbotonal Strategy, most hearing children do not need wireless systems because their binaural listening skills have been fully developed. The goal is to mainstream them with their binaural hearing aids or monaural cochlear implant with monaural hearing aid. This binaural amplification allows each child to blend into the mainstream environment without drawing attention to the fact that they are different. The school audiologist evaluates if a wireless system is needed, and provides an appropriate system when it will contribute to the child's success. The wireless system may be a necessary accommodation in the IEP.

Some children will need a wireless system to be good listeners in the noisy classroom; however, all middle school teenagers are sensitive about looking exactly like their peers in the normal-hearing group. Most of these children will reject a wireless system during this period of their lives because it makes them look different. Their fear is that their peers will not accept them; therefore, the goal is to make each child an effective binaural listener through only their binaural aids. This is the safest and most acceptable way for a the teenager.

Error Analysis

The clinician uses error analysis with the seven parameters to establish good rhythm and intonation speech patterns. At the sentence level, she also uses phoneme analysis to identify the omissions and substitutions in the child's speech patterns. Table 6–6 displays three examples of typical errors that need correction (A. Dowell, personal communication, 2005). The first column is what the child produces, the second column is the target sentences, and the third column is an analysis of errors. The clinician needs to correct these errors as soon as possible, using the child's listening skills. Intelligible speech patterns are necessary for successful mainstreaming.

Table 6–6. Example of Error Analyses

Child Said	Correct Phrase/Sentence	Summary of Mistakes
I wan do doe.	I want to go.	Omission of final /t/ in "want" Substitution of /d/ for /t/ in "to" Substitution of /d/ for /g/ in "go"
My mommy nah here.	My mommy is not here.	Omission of "is" Omission of final /t/ in "not"
I nah ha dat.	I do not have that.	Omission of "do" Omission of final /t/ in "not" Omission of /v/ in "have" Substitution of /d/ for /th/ in "that"

Treatment of Special Populations

Introduction

The Verbotonal Hearing and Speech Center (SUVAG Polyclinic) in Zagreb, Croatia provides Verbotonal Treatment for all types of speech and hearing disorders. Using a medical-educational model, Professor Peter Guberina created the Verbotonal Center in 1954. Physicians of all specialties work closely with speech and hearing specialists at the Center. This approach is used to treat approximately 800 clients per day, which range from very young children to elderly adults in either individual or group treatment sessions.

The Verbotonal Auditory Training Unit is used with all the special populations; for example, articulation speech disorders are corrected while listening through an octave filter. The Verbotonal Approach utilizes all the treatment tools described earlier in this book, for example, vestibular exercises, body movements, the seven speech parameters, nursery rhymes, situational teaching, phonemic progression, suprasegmental tests, tonality tests, amd so forth.

The Center also has a large Verbotonal Foreign Language Program, offering the development of spoken language in seven different languages. In short, the Center utilizes the Verbotonal Approach for all these populations of speech disorders and speech differences. The next section describes how the Verbotonal strategy is applied to some of these different populations in the United States.

Assessment

A comprehensive assessment is obtained before implementing the Verbotonal Strategy. One special assessment is to evaluate the child's vestibular system for possible balance and space perception problems. Children who have a vestibular weakness begin with vestibular exercises.

Other children who have multiple handicaps have a poorer prognosis, because it takes them longer to develop their spoken language skills. Their treatment program needs to be designed to meet their specific needs. In all cases the Individual Education Plan (IEP) is developed with the assistance of a multidisciplinary team and the parent(s).

Hearing Impairment and Deafness

Children who have a mild, moderate, or severe hearing impairment (25 dB to 89 dB HL), immediately benefit from vibrotactile speech input and binaural headsets. Their listening skills develop within one year of daily treatment (1,000 hours) with good rhythm and intonation speech patterns. Their speech intelligibility is dependent on the level of their listening skills.

The children who are profoundly deaf (+90 dB HL), take longer to achieve the same spoken language skills. Their low-frequency residual hearing is usually 20 to 30 dB better than their average hearing loss of 90 dB HL. For example, their pure-tone thresholds at 125 Hz and 250 Hz may be 60 to 70 dB HL. The low-frequency residual hearing can be stimulated with the broad bandwidth (2 to 20,000 Hz) of the Verbotonal Auditory Training Unit. The vibrotactile speech input and the binaural headsets provide this extended low speech frequency stimulation. Maximizing their low-frequency speech perception allows them to also develop good listening skills to self-correct their speech errors.

Auditory Processing Disorders

Children with auditory processing disorders (APD) have normal pure-tone sensitivity but have problems processing spoken language. Some of the children have unintelligible speech patterns and have difficulty imitating speech rhymes, because they have a short-term memory problem.

Over the past 30 years, Knox County Schools have identified these children by three years of age and assigned them to the class of children who have a hearing impairment. For example, a class of three-year-olds may have six children with hearing impairments and two children with normal pure-tone hearing sensitivity. The common element of the class is that all of the children have difficulty processing spoken language. To help them process it, the Verbotonal Auditory Training Unit is used simultaneously with the binaural headset and vibrotactile speech input. The most comfortable loudness level (MCL) of the clinician's voice is adjusted for each child in each earphone. For example, a child with a profound hearing loss of 90 dB HL would have the speech input set for 110 dB SPL, and the child with normal pure-tone sensitivity has it set for 65 dB SPL. The children use their most comfortable loudness level to process the clinician's speech input.

The clinician utilizes all the Verbotonal treatment tools—vestibular exercises, body movements, the seven speech parameters, phonemic progression, nursery rhymes, situational teaching, and so forth. Even though these eight children have different levels of hearing sensitivity, the individual MCL levels help them imitate the clinician's speech model. An independent observer would conclude that all eight of the children have a hearing impairment, because they have a similar speech output and the same strategy is used for each child.

The children with normal pure-tone sensitivity progress more quickly than the children with a hearing impairment. The daily speech stimulation through headsets and vibrotactile speech input provides an optimum learning condition for them to progress at a fast rate. Usually, after one year of daily speech stimulation (1,000 hours per year), these children can be mainstreamed into a regular preschool or a kindergarten class. Both their speech patterns and their auditory processing skills are within the normal range. The daily intensive auditory-based stimulation allows them to progress quickly. Knox County Schools have provided the Verbotonal treatment for the past 30 years (1975–present), and it has been very successful.

Another type of auditory processing disorder are children who are having academic difficulty in elementary school. Typically, these children have difficulty following the directions of the classroom teacher, and this makes it difficult for them to complete their academic assignments. These children have normal intelligence and have been diagnosed as having an auditory processing disorder.

In private practice, a Verbotonal clinician worked for ten years implementing the Verbotonal Strategy to improve each child's auditory processing skills (L. Rook, personal communication, 2005). She used the Verbotonal Auditory Training Unit by setting the low-pass filter, for example, 500 Hz, to emphasize the listening to rhythm and intonation patterns. Once the children can imitate an entire speech rhyme, for example, "Ah Boo, Bah Boo, Boo Boo, Bah Boo," their short-term memory span was better. She also uses written symbols for nonsense syllable speech rhymes to expand their memory span. Seeing the written symbols helped the children structure their memory span. After daily individual treatment sessions of one hour for three months, these children demonstrated an improvement in their academic performance. The clinician also applied these Verbotonal treatment techniques in Knox County Schools. She was able to obtain the same good results in school that she did in private practice (Rook, 2005). The following is a description of the treatment tools she used for the suprasegmentals, fading auditory memory, and decoding of spoken language.

The adaptability of the Verbotonal Approach has been shown frequently and successfully over the past several years when the treatment tools and strategies have been applied to children and adults diagnosed with auditory processing disorder (APD). As with clients who are hearing impaired, the primary areas of focus during the initial stages of treatment are: (1) the suprasegmentals of spoken language,

(2) the auditory memory (fading memory), and (3) the decoding of phonemes in less than optimal listening conditions (Rook, 2005).

1. Suprasegmentals

Many audiologists, speech pathologist, and hearing clinicians have observed that a significant number of patients tested for auditory processing difficulties seem to have difficulty when general movements and vocalizations are attempted simultaneously. It is difficult for them to repeat simple monosyllabic patterns with the same rhythm and stress (intensity) as the clinician's model. In severe cases, it may be difficult for the client to reproduce the length of utterance (duration), that is, producing a long versus short "bah" after the clinician presents the speech model. If an unstressed element in a syllable pattern becomes too "short" for the client to hear, he or she may omit the syllable altogether when attempting to repeat the pattern. One quickly realizes the impact of not hearing or perceiving unstressed elements in everyday speech on a listener's auditory comprehension (Rook, 2005).

The use of body movements as a treatment tool has been shown to be an effective means of enabling the client to simultaneously hear, feel, and see the suprasegmentals of speech. Through stimulating and corrective movements, a clinician can visually and kinesthetically portray the elements of tension, pitch, timing, duration, and stress for all vocalizations. The clinician can modify the client's perception and production of speech by changing her body movement after analyzing the client's speech error and imitative movements (Rook, 2005).

Another observation made frequently by skilled clinicians analyzing the spontaneous or imitative speech of many children diagnosed with APD is the lack of intonation, or pitch variation, in their vocalizations. These clients may sound monotonal and lack expression in their speech. If one accepts the premise that individuals produce speech in the manner in which they perceive it (e.g., dialect differences), then it is important to determine whether the client can perceive the intonation changes and if he has the ability to produce a wider range of pitch changes in his speech (Rook, 2005).

2. Fading Auditory Memory

The fading auditory memory of the client with APD is targeted as a critical area of remediation from the onset of treatment. This is due to the tremendous impact that memory has upon the entire ability to process auditory information with speed and accuracy. A clinician must strengthen the client's ability to "hold" the amount of auditory information for the length of time necessary for the information to be retained. The ability to concentrate for several minutes at a time also can be positively impacted by treatment strategies that are designed to strengthen the client's fading auditory memory (Rook, 2005).

When developing or strengthening fading auditory memory, a clinician must be careful to design activities that are primarily auditory in presentation. The client's responses must be analyzed by what he heard and remembered the clinician saying, not by what he saw in terms of therapy materials or movements. For example, the clinician puts four sequencing picture cards on the table in front of the client in incorrect order of sequence. The instructions are to listen to four sentences, each one describing a picture. After listening to all the sentences, the client is to put the pictures in the same order in which the sentences were produced. If the client has a normal visual memory, he may simply look at the pictures as the clinician speaks and make a mental note of which picture is number 1, 2, 3, and 4. Then, he can easily put the pictures in order because he remembers each picture's position, not necessarily remembering what he heard. A more effective way of strengthening fading memory would be to say the four sentences prior to showing the pictures. The client would then have to "hold" the information heard while he searches for the correct picture. This increased amount of holding time strengthens both memory and focusing skills (Rook, 2005).

Most clinicians will agree that it is easier for clients to remember auditory information when it is presented as meaningful language. Therefore, using nonlinguistic auditory input, unrelated single words and numbers, and nonsense segmental patterns in treatment can be more effective than language-based activities. Even visual information, particularly when used with suprasegmental and fading memory training, may be abstract in nature and have no conceptual content. The clinician may use voice modification techniques, such as altering the rhythm, stress, intonation, or pause between elements to cue the client to enable him to remember more of the auditory stimuli for a greater length of time (Rook, 2005).

A strategy that has been effective in developing the auditory memory and suprasegmental perception of the APD client is the use of cards, which visually portray the suprasegmental qualities of speech. For example, rhythm cards have a series of dots and dashes to symbolize the duration of sounds. A series of dots and dashes represent rhythm patterns that become progressively longer and more difficult to remember. The clinician can use these cards in numerous ways depending on the needs of the client (Rook, 2005).

Each rhythm card has between three and seven syllables for a duration, intonation, or loudness pattern. For example, a 4-syllable duration pattern might be a short-short-short-long pattern. An intonation pattern might be upward-downward-upward-downward, and a loudness pattern might be loud-soft-soft-loud. Each rhythm card is marked clearly, so the client can use his visual memory to repeat back each auditory pattern. Later, the client can repeat back the auditory pattern, without seeing the visual rhythm cards.

3. Decoding

The decoding of the phonemes of the English language can be difficult, especially if the client struggles to decode or perceive the suprasegmentals of duration, pitch, intensity, tension, and word frequency. The client should be trained during the initial stages of treatment to discriminate and reproduce the differences in the intensity, length, speed, and the pitch and frequency of the phonemes. He should also be aware of and able to imitate the tension and placement variations of phonemes. Discrimination of phonemes, sound blending, articulation of phonemes, processing time, and sequencing are all processing skills that can be enhanced by using Verbotonal strategies. Body movements facilitate the perception and production of sounds (in isolation or in patterns), phonetic rhymes or nonsense rhythms help to develop good memory and sequencing skills, and filtered listening (Verbotonal Auditory Training Unit) trains the client to perceive speech when it is presented to him in limited frequency bands, therefore enabling him to hear better in noise and to comprehend spoken language more efficiently when auditory information is limited (auditory closure) (Rook, 2005).

Articulation Disorders

The Verbotonal Strategy for children with articulation disorders involves using binaural headsets of the Verbotonal Auditory Training Unit to attenuate the room noise by 30 dB and pass the optimal octave for the target phoneme. For example, to correct a /ʃ/ substitution error for the target /s/ phoneme, the octave filter is set at a center frequency of 6000 Hz. The octave filter eliminates the frequencies of the child's error (e.g., /ʃ/ substitution at 4000 Hz). Once the child can correctly perceive the target sound, he can self-correct his errors in conversational speech with carryover to everyday situations.

If needed, the optimal octave filter can be adjusted as higher or lower in frequency to make a greater perceptual separation of the target phoneme and the substitution error. For example, the optimal octave is moved to 8000 Hz center frequency to obtain a 4000 Hz separation (4000 Hz = /ʃ/ and 8000 Hz = /s/). This greater separation is necessary for some children to refine their speech discrimination skills to produce a sharper /s/ sound.

The next procedure is to add a low-pass filter of 300 Hz to provide the rhythm and intonation patterns of the target sound in a word or phrase; for example, "Sally is sick." If the target sound is correct in this spoken phrase, then the training unit is changed from an octave filter to a wideband listening condition. The wideband listening helps the child adjust to an everyday listening situation. Carryover is evaluated by having the child listen without the headset. This is the final stage of carryover in the treatment session.

The Verbotonal procedure was tested in the Knox County Public Schools with a research grant. A group of children with articulation disorders were pretested with the *Goldman-Fristoe Test of Articulation* on 73 single phonemes and phoneme blends. The children varied in the number of errors, ranging from 3 to 23 errors out of a possible 73 test items. There was an average of 15 errors for the whole group. The Verbotonal strategy described above was used for two 30-minute individual treatment sessions per week. The average treatment time was 11.5 hours for the group. The post-test scores indicated that the group had decreased from an average of 15 errors to an average of 8 errors and that the children needed an average of 2 hours of treatment to correct each error. The school speech-language pathologist, who later worked with the same children, reported that these children had better speech discrimination skills and better carryover than children who underwent a traditional treatment approach.

A second part of this research project applied the same Verbotonal strategy to a normal-hearing group of preschoolers who had severe language and articulation delay. The pretest of the 73 phonemes and blends showed an average of 60 errors. After the Verbotonal treatment, the average number of errors decreased to 30 out of the 73 test items. The preschoolers actually showed greater progress than the elementary school children. The octave filter was more effective for the younger children.

In Miami-Dade County Schools, the Verbotonal clinicians were assigned children with articulation disorders and normal hearing as part of their caseload. The clinicians applied the octave filter treatment described above to these children. They reported a significant improvement in the children's performance when listening through the optimal octave filter. Most of these children were dismissed from treatment, because their articulation errors were corrected.

As explained earlier, the Verbotonal Center in Zagreb, Croatia uses the optimal octave filter for all their children with articulation disorders.

The Verbotonal clinicians' rationale is that the headsets with the octave filters help the children correct their misarticulations by listening. Carryover to conversational speech can then occur.

The Verbotonal strategy described above is different from a traditional speech strategy. The traditional speech pathologist uses a stimulus-response model that uses the same target model without a speech modification based on the child's error(s). The assumption is that the child will correct himself if he hears the target model often enough. The traditional clinician may use phonetic placement with a mirror to show the child how to place his tongue in the proper position for articulating the sound. The assumption is that if the child understands where to place his tongue, he will be able to correct his speech error.

In contrast to the traditional clinician, the Verbotonal clinician assumes that the child's error occurs because the child does not auditorally perceive the target phoneme correctly. Therefore, optimal octave filters are used so the child can perceive the sound correctly and adjust his tongue position without any visual cues from the clinician or visual feedback through a mirror.

As normal coarticulation patterns are the goal of all clinicians, it seems most logical to correct through auditory perception. This way the child can make the necessary articulatory adjustments to produce the target phonemes in a variety of phoneme environments. The auditory-based strategy of the Verbotonal Approach provides a better framework for the child to have successful carryover to a variety of conversational contexts.

Language Disorders

The Verbotonal Strategy for children with mild or severe language disorders is the same as the strategy described earlier for the children with hearing impairments. The children with severe language disorder need intensive intervention at the preschool age level. Most of these children are classified as having a learning disability. Their verbal test scores are below average, even though their nonverbal intelligence quotient (NVIQ) is within the normal range. Some of these children may have an attention deficit disorder (ADD or ADHD), which makes it very difficult for them to concentrate and learn in traditional programs. The binaural headsets of the Verbotonal Auditory Training Unit helps these children to focus on the auditory-based input. Some of these children also benefit from vibrotactile speech input. Both input modalities assist the child in concentrating on the clinician's speech model and understanding spoken language. Children with severe language disorders can be placed in a classroom with hearing-impaired children that receive daily stimulation throughout the school year (e.g., 1,000 hours per year).

Children with severe language disorder are difficult to separate from the children who have an auditory processing disorder. Both groups usually experience difficulty imitating speech rhymes and using their auditory memory to process speech input.

Multicultural Populations

The United States is becoming a multicultural society, with many different languages spoken in homes. For example, Miami-Dade County Schools has a large number of Hispanic immigrants, who attend public schools. In many cases, the parents speak Spanish in the home and use minimal English when communicating with their children.

Since American English is the primary language spoken in the public schools, these Hispanic children often have difficulty learning from English textbooks. There is a mismatch between the language used in the home and the language used in the school. This creates problems for these children.

To solve this problem of mismatch, there is a need for bilingual Verbotonal clinicians, who are fluent in both English and Spanish. Bilingual instruction helps the Hispanic children learn about both languages and their use, and both cultures.

Speech Disorder Versus Speech Difference

Speech disorders are usually diagnosed using standardized tests that provide normative data for American English-speaking children. A diagnosed speech disorder is based on the child having speech patterns that deviate from the standardized norms. These children need intervention as soon as possible.

Children with a speech difference use different dialect than Standard American English. These dialect patterns are usually a result of different speech patterns being modeled in the home as compared to those presented in school. It is possible for these children to learn both "home-talk" and "school-talk" and be proficient in both; whereas children with a language disorder are not capable of learning language without treatment intervention.

The Verbotonal clinician needs a thorough understanding of dialect differences and how these differences affect the child at home and in the school environment. She begins by making the child aware of the differences in "home-talk" and "school-talk." These children need to become skilled in the language used in school so that they can learn the curriculum without interference of misunderstanding the language.

At the same time, these bidialectical children can continue to use their "home-talk" with their family; it is equally important to maintain the cultural dialect of these children. The Verbotonal clinician must be able to distinguish between a speech disorder and a speech difference, and provide direct intervention to children with disorders and facilitate language development with children with language differences.

Second Language Learning

Chapter 5 explained the Verbotonal strategy for learning to speak a second language. As most of the Verbotonal clinician's in the United States are English-speaking, they are capable of teaching English as a second language. For example, in Miami-Dade County Schools, there are a large number of children who speak Spanish as their native language. Most of these children immigrated to the United States and immediately enrolled in a public school.

The Verbotonal clinician is well-prepared to teach English as a second language in group treatment. The group treatment can include the film strips and books that were discussed in chapter 5. Initially, these group sessions would be daily, intensive treatment preferably implemented early in the school day. This intensive spoken English stimulation prepares the children for the English speech patterns that the teacher uses in the classroom. Gradually, the Spanish-speaking children transition to using spoken English in the classroom.

For children who are having difficulty making the transition from their native language to spoken English, the Verbotonal clinician should provide individual treatment sessions daily. Both group and individual treatment help the children make a successful transition to speaking the English language.

The Verbotonal treatment is most successful with preschool and elementary school children. In general, the younger the child, the easier it is for them to adjust from spoken Spanish to spoken English. For the older high school students, the treatment sessions need to be held over a longer period of time and the children need to be assigned to an English "buddy" who can help by translating in the classroom.

The Verbotonal strategies can also be used for teaching a variety of foreign languages. The teacher must be trained in the Verbotonal strategy, so that she can use the auditory-based techniques effectively while teaching. As explained in chapter 5, the filmstrips and book that apply to each foreign language help the child progress through the stages of learning a new language and help him to speak fluently. The foreign language teacher should be a native speaker of the language he or she teaches. Ideally, these foreign language courses begin in elementary school; the earlier a new language is introduced, the easier it is for the child to successfully master the language. However, most school systems only offer foreign language instruction in middle school and high school programs.

The important point is that the children can become proficient at speaking in the foreign language. The goal is to make them sound like a native speaker. For example, when the student visits a Spanish-speaking event, the native Spanish speakers will identify him as a native speaker. When this occurs, the foreign language instruction approach has successfully prepared the child for fitting into another culture.

The ability to read in a foreign language develops later and is based on the level of proficiency with which the child speaks the language. The general rule is that speaking skills precede reading skills.

Summary of Special Populations

This section on special populations has described how the Verbotonal Strategy can be applied to a variety of communication disorders. The original model was the Verbotonal Hearing and Speech Center in Zagreb, Croatia. This same model can be used in the United States, even in a public school system. Using the same Verbotonal Strategy allows the clinician to specialize in these treatment tools and to apply them to different populations. The common element in these populations is that most of the children began with unintelligible speech and poor listening skills. This is the feature that allows one treatment strategy to be used for different disorders.

Treatment of Adults

Introduction

The Verbotonal Hearing and Speech Center (SUVAG Polyclinic) in Zagreb, Croatia is the Model Center that provides treatment for adults with a hearing impairment. The Center serves more than 50 adults each day for treatment (auditory training) and hearing aid placement. The treatment involves six individual treatment rooms, with each room equipped with a Verbotonal Auditory Training Unit. Each Verbotonal clinician uses binaural headsets and auditory speech input to develop the clients' auditory brain transfer in the low-frequency speech zone. Each client completes three 30-minute treatment sessions per week to improve auditory speech perception, for example, to improve from a 40% speech recognition to 80% recognition. The treatment sessions continue until an 80% speech recognition is achieved, or the client stops improving. This treatment is usually completed in one to three months.

In the United States, this treatment model is difficult to implement because most Americans want a "quick fix" with a wearable hearing aid. However, the Blount Hearing and Speech Center in Maryville, Tennessee uses the Zagreb Model. Clients who have a low speech recognition score (e.g., 40%) are referred to auditory training treatment before hearing aid placement occurs.

An explanation of auditory training for adults precedes hearing aid placement because the auditory strategy is needed to fully understand the success of proper hearing aid placement. The reader is encouraged to review how the acoustic filters are used (see chapter 3).

The Need for Treatment for Adults

The number of adults with a hearing impairment is greater than 10% of the United States population. This percentage increases each year because people are living longer. In comparison, the number of children with profound hearing loss is less than 1% of the population.

Hearing loss has an immediate impact on the communication skills of young children. This is because the children have not yet developed the auditory or verbal skills necessary for verbal communication; instead they have unintelligible speech and poor listening skills. Federal and State legislation mandates that services be provided for these children immediately.

In contrast, adults with a hearing impairment do not receive the same attention as children. Some adults with hearing loss do not research or seek the services that are available to them. In these cases a spouse, family member, or friend must insist that the individual seek out these services. Most adults have an acquired hearing loss that develops gradually over time. One cause is associated with the high noise level of the environment, and this excess noise is increasing each year, especially in large, developed cites. In addition to the overall noise of the environment, other types of excess noise exist within the workplace and in recreational activities. For example, noise-induced hearing loss is very common in noisy factories. These adults have what is called a Carhardt notch, which is a 40 dB to 70 dB hearing loss centered mostly at 4000 Hz.

Most of these adults have difficulty understanding speech in a noisy environment, because the noise masks or interferes with the low-frequency speech recognition. These adults are usually considered hard-of-hearing, with most of their hearing loss above 1000 Hz. Their hearing sensitivity below 1000 Hz can actually be near or close to normal hearing (25 dB HL).

In most cases, the adults retain their normal speech patterns, even though they have a hearing loss. This is very different from the unintelligible speech patterns of children with hearing loss. The normal speech patterns of adults are a result of their normal proprioceptive memory patterns. In short, these memory patterns allow them to retain normal speech even though they have difficulty hearing themselves speak. Their low-frequency sensitivity provides sufficient auditory feedback along with their proprioceptive memory span.

Because most of these adults have intelligible speech, the identification of their hearing loss may go undetected. It is often the spouse, family member, or friend who interacts with the individual on a regular basis that can detect the effects of hearing loss on the individual's communication skills. The lack of communication skills can become so bad that they avoid normal communication situations. This withdrawal attitude has a negative effect on their emotional and psychological well-being.

Recent advances in technology has made wearing hearing aids and/or cochlear implants more useful and practical. For example, hearing aids are now available in analog or digital technology, with advanced microphone sensitivity and placement. Considering these advancements, it should be possible to achieve great success in hearing aid placement. Unfortunately, this is not the case; more than 50% of adults who have hearing aids are not satisfied with them. Some are so dissatisfied with their functioning, especially in noisy environments, that they permanently discontinue their use. This represents a high percent (50%) of failure with using hearing aids to minimize the effects of hearing loss on communication skills. The Verbotonal strategy offers a solution to this problem, whereby more adults with hearing impairment can be helped. The next section describes this strategy.

Auditory Brain Transfer

In order to help children and/or adults with a hearing impairment, the Verbotonal clinician must understand auditory brain transfer. There are two types of auditory brain transfer: one is natural transfer and the other is treatment transfer. In both types the neuroplasticity of the client's brain allows the brain to restructure its neural connections to the cochlea, so that the low-frequency zone processes both low and high-frequency speech energy. This allows the client to make maximum use of his residual hearing in the low-frequency zone.

One way to understand auditory brain transfer is to describe how a client with hearing impairment developed "natural" transfer. For example, the writer of this book had a teenager client with a "ski-slope" hearing loss. The client had normal pure-tone thresholds of 15 dB from 125 Hz to 1000 Hz. Then, at 2000 Hz to 8000 Hz, he had a profound hearing loss. When the client was tested with tonality sentences and tonality words, he had speech recognition scores of 100%. The tonality sentences were easier than the words; he immediately repeated the sentences correctly. For the high-tonality words, the client delayed some with his response, but was eventually able to repeat the words correctly. The client's high level of performance was achieved without any visual cues; he was not able to see the clinician's facial expressions. He could only hear the tonality sentences and words at a most comfortable loudness level.

Next, a binaural headset from the Verbotonal Auditory Training Unit was placed on the client. The low-pass filter was set at (0) 1000 Hz (60). All of the speech frequencies below 1000 Hz were passed naturally, and all speech frequencies above 1000 Hz were eliminated (attenuated). This particular client was able to perceive both low and high speech frequencies within the low-frequency zone (below 1000 Hz). This individual's brain had naturally developed low-frequency speech transfer and scored 100% on speech recognition without any visual cues. All clients have the possibility to develop "natural" brain transfer; however, depending on the pure-tone configuration and the type of hearing loss, some clients only develop a small amount of brain transfer. The Verbotonal clinician should evaluate his client's auditory speech perception to see how much brain transfer has been developed naturally.

In 1966, Rhodes documented natural auditory brain transfer by testing the speech recognition of adults with normal hearing and adults with a "ski-slope" hearing loss at 1000 Hz. He tested their speech recognition by passing the speech test input through a 1000 Hz low-pass filter. The adults with a hearing impairment scored 18% higher (59% vs. 31%) than those with normal hearing. He wrote that the adults with hearing impairment had learned to compensate by utilizing the low-frequency zone to compensate for their high-frequency hearing loss. He concluded that adults with a hearing impairment learned to use low-frequency cues that adults with normal hearing do not usually use. The fact that the adult with the hearing impairment can outperform normal-hearing adults is amazing and demonstrates the brain's neuroplasticity.

The second type of brain transfer is developed through the Verbotonal Treatment Strategy. This treatment involves intensive 30-minute sessions of listening practice, with the acoustic filters set for the optimal frequency response. The treatment for perceptual transfer will be explained later in this chapter.

Pre-Hearing Aid Assessment

Before designing a treatment plan for auditory training, the Verbotonal clinician completes a comprehensive Pre-Hearing Aid Assessment. Table 6–7 identifies the areas of this assessment. To establish a baseline for comparison, the client's unaided (no hearing aid) auditory speech perception is evaluated first (see Table 6–7). Based on the client's

Table 6–7. Verbotonal Pre-Hearing Aid Assessment

1. Unaided: No Hearing Aid	
Best Tonality Zone Hz	ft. Best Distance
2. Aided: Hearing Aid(s): Best Zone Hz	
or Cochlear Implant	% at 15 feet
3. Verbotonal Training Unit: Bin. Headsets	
a. Optimal Frequency Response (OFR)	
• Transfer	Yes/No
• SRT Line	Hz
• SRT/SDT Difference	dB
b. Speech Tempo (Normal = 5 syllabls/second)	Syllable/second
c. Dynamic Range (Normal = +20 dB)	
• UL-MCL	dB
d. Signal/Noise Ratio (Normal = 5 dB)	dB
e. Reverbation (Normal = 1.8 Rev. Time)	RT
4. Vibrotactile Speech Input	%
5. Speech Intelligibility	%
6. Tinnitus (Masked by OFR)	Yes/No

pure-tone thresholds and speech reception thresholds, the Fletcher Unaided Graph is used to estimate the client's optimal unaided listening distance for each ear. The "better" ear is evaluated first, with the poorer ear plugged. This was explained in detail in chapter 3.

As a comparison, an adult with normal hearing can understand speech at distances greater than 30 feet. In contrast, an adult with a speech reception threshold (SRT) of 55 dB should understand speech at a distance of 3 feet, and an adult with an SRT of 85 dB would only understand speech at a distance of 1 inch or less. This unaided distance is measured from the clinician's mouth to the listener's ear.

This optimum unaided distance is equivalent to the client's most comfortable loudness level. Once this distance is established, the clinician presents a Tonality Word Test without any visual cues. The result of this test identifies the tonality zone of best perception for the client. For example, a test score of 80% for both the low and the low-middle zones indicate that these zones are the optimal tonality zones; whereas, a score of 10% for the high zone indicates that the high-tonality zone is not ideal for the client. After the "better" ear is tested, the same testing procedures are applied to the "poorer" ear, with an earplug or masking noise in the better ear. For this client, let us assume that his "better" unaided tonality score is 50% at a distance of 3 feet. If the client is already using a hearing aid(s), the same test procedure is also performed with the hearing aid(s) in place. The aided tonality test is performed at a standard distance of 15 feet. Let us assume the client's overall tonality score is 30%; this indicates that the client's aided score is worse than his unaided score of 50%. These results suggest that the client is not obtaining the maximum benefit from his hearing aid(s).

The next phase of assessment involves the binaural headset of the Verbotonal Auditory Training Unit (Table 6–7). The optimal frequency response is based on the best tonality zone of the unaided evaluation and the SRT line from the client's audiogram. For example, the frequency zone of 125 to 1000 Hz is the optimal frequency zone for the client's "better" ear. Using the optimal zone (e.g., (0) 1000 (60)), a series of assessment tests are completed.

The first test is a speech tempo test (Table 6–7). The clinician speaks "tonality sentences" at a normal speech rate of five syllables per second. If the client performs poorly, she slows her rate to 2 syllables per second. If the client achieves better scores (% correct) with the slower rate, this suggests that the client has difficulty with the normal rate/tempo of speech.

Next, the clinician compares the client's most comfortable loudness (MCL) with the uncomfortable loudness level (UCL) for tonality sentences. If the difference between these levels is less than 20 dB (e.g.,

MCL = 70 dB and UCL = 80 dB), the client has significant recruitment (decreased loudness tolerance) for speech.

In the next assessment, the clinician evaluates the client's tolerance for competing noise. If the client can only understand tonality sentences with +15 dB S/N ratio, then he has difficulty with competing noise. The clinician then adds reverberation to the speech input to evaluate the client's speech perception with reverberation under the headset. If the client cannot tolerate reverberation of 1.8 seconds, then he has reduced auditory perception when reverberation is added.

In the example above, the client has a reduced tolerance for the following: normal speech tempo, dynamic range, S/N ratio, and reverberation. These results suggest that the client needs auditory training treatment to improve his speech recognition under all these conditions. Ideally, the auditory training treatment is completed before the hearing aid(s) is placed.

For further evaluation, the vibrotactile speech input is added to the binaural headset input to evaluate whether this added input improves his speech perception. If the client does improve, the vibrator is always used as part of the optimal frequency response.

Then, the client's speech intelligibility is evaluated. If the client has 100% speech intelligibility, no special treatment is needed; however if speech intelligibility is less than 80%, the treatment plan should include developing listening skills to correct speech errors.

The client is also evaluated for possible tinnitus, or ringing in the ear(s). The clinician presents the optimal frequency response through the filters to mask the client's tinnitus. If this is successful, his prognosis is good; however, if the filters do not mask the tinnitus, the client has a poorer prognosis for improving his speech recognition.

In summary, Table 6–7 provides a comprehensive list of functional tests for the Pre-Hearing Aid Assessment. These assessment procedures are important for developing an effective auditory training treatment plan.

Adverse Listening Conditions

Elementary school children, who have completed the Preschool and School-Age Verbotonal Treatment, are similar to adults with a mild-to-moderate hearing loss. Both the children and the adults have intelligible spoken language. They are also similar in that their auditory speech recognition is at least 80% correct. Both the children and the adults needed improvement in their speech recognition in noise and reverberation. This involved changing the optimal learning condition to an adverse learning condition. To accomplish this, noise and reverberation were added through the Verbotonal Auditory Training Unit. For example, the S/N ratio is +5 dB and the reverberation time is 1.0 seconds. The adverse listening condition allows both children and adults to practice their speech recognition in a condition that approximates the everyday listening conditions that are difficult for them. By practicing under adverse conditions, they are able to make improvements in their speech recognition in the presence of noise.

Verbotonal Auditory Training for Adults

The Verbotonal Auditory Training is similar for adults and elementary school children, but to simplify the discussion, the training is described for adults. The Verbotonal treatment strategies should be applied as needed and when appropriate. The Verbotonal Auditory Training Unit, with the binaural headsets and vibrotactile speech input, is the main treatment tool.

The test results from the Pre-Hearing Aid Assessment are used to plan an intensive auditory training program. The optimal frequency response is obtained by having the client repeat sentences as the clinician adjusts the low-pass filter. The clinician begins with a (6) 1000 (60) Hz setting. The 6 dB slope toward the low frequencies gradually attenuates some of the low-frequency speech energy. If this initial setting is not optimal, the clinician switches to a 0 dB slope to allow more of the low-frequency speech energy. The 60 dB slope toward the high frequencies is a sharp slope to reduce the mid-to-high and high-frequency zones. This allows the clinician to avoid the area of the greatest hearing loss, which usually results in some perceptual distortion. For some clients, the addition of a high-pass filter at 2000 Hz or 4000 Hz is helpful. If this is the case, the filter is placed near or at the client's threshold. This occurs when the low-frequency speech energy makes the client more sensitive to some high speech frequencies at his or her threshold. This is considered an optimal bimodal listening condition. Feedback from the adult client is used to evaluate these filter settings to arrive at the optimal frequency response.

The clinician obtains additional information by comparing the results of the best tonality zone of the unaided test condition with the aided test condition. The clinician also draws a speech reception threshold (SRT) line on the client's audiogram to help identify the best tonality zone for the client.

A comparison between the SRT and the speech detection threshold (SDT) also provides important information. If the difference between these two values is 5 dB or less, it suggests that the client can perceive speech information through the low-frequency zone and that he has successfully developed brain transfer through the low-frequency zone.

Using the optimal frequency response, the clinician conducts a series of 30-minute auditory training sessions. The clinician instructs the client to repeat short and/or long sentences that are of the same general topic (e.g., holiday, recent event, etc.). This allows the client to be more successful in speech recognition. If needed, the clinician adjusts her speech tempo from a normal rate (5 syllables per second) to a slow rate (2 syllables per second).

If the client is successful with both the slow and normal rate, the clinician can present speech at a faster rate (8 syllables per second) for additional practice. If the client successfully perceives all the words correctly without any visual cues, the speech tempo practice has been effective.

To practice dynamic range, the client's SRT is lowered until there is a 20+ dB difference between the SRT and the Uncomfortable Loudness Level (UCL). This is accomplished by gradually reducing the speech input level presented through the binaural headsets as the client repeats short and long sentences. With a few practice sessions, most clients are able to maintain a high speech recognition, even though the speech level has been lowered (e.g., 65 dB HL to 55 dB HL). An increase in dynamic range usually helps to minimize recruitment (an abnormal growth in loudness). A dynamic range that is greater than 20 dB allows the client to be more successful hearing aid users.

The assessment of signal-to-noise ratio is used to determine the settings for the Verbotonal Auditory Training Unit. The clinician begins with a +15 dB S/N ratio, which is an easy listening condition for most clients. She gradually increases the level of noise while the client repeats familiar sentences, allowing the client to practice in an adverse listening condition. Once the client is able to repeat the sentences at +5 dB or 0 dB S/N ratio, he is able to maintain his speech recognition score of at least 80% in the presence of noise.

The amount of reverberation presented with the speech input is adjusted on the training unit, beginning at a low level of 0.6 seconds and increasing to a high level of 1.8 seconds. Once the client can repeat sentences without being distracted by the reverberation, he is able to maintain a high level of speech recognition at different reverberation times.

Finally, all the adverse practice conditions are presented simultaneously (e.g., 0 dB S/N ratio and 1.8 second reverberation time). A client that has reached this level of success is a good candidate for hearing aid placement.

If the client has poor speech intelligibility, the clinician corrects the speech errors in the optimal frequency response condition. This correction strategy uses error analysis of the seven speech parameters. For example, increasing the duration of the /s/ consonant while adding a high-frequency filter at 6000 Hz usually helps the client perceive the /s/ correctly.

Auditory training is also used to reduce or eliminate the client's tinnitus. The filter of the training unit is adjusted to the ringing in the client's ears. For example, a 2000 Hz filter might mask the client's tinnitus, and thus reduce the negative effects the ringing has on the repeating sentences task.

Through all this training, the clinician's goal is to maximize the client's auditory brain transfer. This happens when the most sensitive low-frequency zone is maximized. The client uses the low zones to perceive both low and high speech frequencies. With practice through an optimal frequency response condition, it is possible for a client to achieve 100% speech recognition through the Verbotonal Auditory Training Unit. The next task is to achieve the same high level of speech recognition through the client's hearing aid(s) or cochlear implant.

Hearing Aid Placement

As described earlier, the Verbotonal Hearing and Speech Center in Zagreb, Croatia requires Verbotonal Auditory Training prior to hearing aid placement. These training sessions must demonstrate a marked improvement in the client's speech recognition when visual cues are minimized. To achieve this higher level of perception, the client must have developed auditory brain transfer.

Under these conditions, Croatia medical insurance will pay for the client's hearing aid. In the United States, adult clients have to pay for their hearing aid(s) themselves. As a result, the Zagreb Hearing Aid Model is difficult to implement in the United States. Often, clients in the United States want to purchase their hearing aid(s) and receive immediate amplification and do not want to put in the time necessary for the auditory training sessions.

The Blount Hearing and Speech Center in Maryville, Tennessee follows the Zagreb Model as closely as possible. The Center completes a pre-hearing aid assessment for each client to determine if auditory training is appropriate. Then, the client must choose to complete the training before the hearing aid placement or to purchase the hearing aid(s) without auditory training.

The owner of the Blount Hearing and Speech Center is Mr. John Berry, a certified Verbotonal clinician. Mr. Berry has 35 years of experience (1970 to present) with using the Verbotonal Approach and treatment tools (Berry, personal communication, 2005). He began by working with preschool children with hearing impairment to develop listening skills and intelligible speech patterns. Later, he developed a Verbotonal Auditory Training Program for adults. Through private practice, he was able to refine the Verbotonal treatment strategies and tools for hearing aid placement. Mr. Berry's Hearing and Speech Center has consistently demonstrated outstanding results with their clients. The Center offers a 100% satisfaction guarantee, or the client's money is refunded. Twenty percent of the clients travel from out-of-state to the center to receive services. This demonstrates the excellent reputation of Mr. Berry's treatment program and his staff that provide the services. He has built his reputation by implementing the strategies and treatment tools of the Verbotonal Approach. The following is a description of how the Blount Center uses the Verbotonal Approach in hearing aid placement.

After the pre-hearing aid assessment has been completed using the Verbotonal Auditory Training Unit, the client decides to enroll in the Auditory Training Program or to purchase a hearing aid(s). With either decision, the Verbotonal clinician selects a hearing aid to fit the client's optimal frequency response. The clinician chooses an aid from the large hearing aid inventory that includes a variety of companies and a variety of models. The clinician frequently selects a hearing aid with an extended low-frequency response with a variety of slopes. This is helpful in following the optimal frequency response of the client.

Mr. Berry follows the principle that the clinician should order the hearing aid that is most appropriate for each individual, considering all applicable characteristics (e.g., gain and frequency response). He feels that the trained Verbotonal clinician is responsible for selecting the most appropriate hearing aid, not the hearing aid companies. This is different from most conventional audiologists, who allow the company to select the hearing aid and specific settings using the test data provided.

The next principle of the Verbotonal approach is to use the information from the pre-hearing aid assessment to estimate the amount of brain transfer that has occurred in the low-frequency zone. This requires the use of a low-pass filter on the Verbotonal Auditory Training Unit or the individual's hearing aid. Using the Tonality Word Test and error analysis of the seven parameters, the clinician can determine the amount of perceptual transfer that has occurred. In other words the clinician can evaluate whether the client is able to use the low-frequency zone to perceive high-frequency speech sounds. This Verbotonal principle is in contrast to the conventional procedure of mirroring the hearing loss, which involves more amplification (gain) of the frequencies of greatest loss (e.g., the high-frequency zone). The goal of providing greater amplification of these high frequencies is to have aided pure-tone thresholds in free field that are flat at 25 dB or less. This means the frequency of 4000 Hz may have a gain (amplification) of 80 dB. In short, this strategy is attempting to amplify the "Dead Frequency Zone(s)." Recent research suggests that these "Dead Frequency Zones" may not be perceptually useful with a 70 dB or greater hearing loss. These zones need to be avoided.

The third principle of the Verbotonal Approach is to use a behind-the-ear model hearing aid whenever possible. This model allows for a more precise adjustment of the earmold. For example, for clients with a "ski-slope" hearing loss, an open or free-field mold is most appropriate, because this type of hearing loss has mild (20–40 dB) thresholds below 1000 Hz and severe-to-profound thresholds above 1000 Hz. With an open, free-field mold, the speech frequencies can pass naturally, without amplification. The clinician uses the Tonality Word Test to evaluate the client's speech recognition at 15 feet. Then, she presents a high-frequency response through the hearing aid to accompany the unamplified low frequencies. This is an effective bimodal presentation, in which only the high frequencies are amplified.

In summary, Mr. John Berry has developed a successful hearing aid placement program based on the Verbotonal treatment strategies and treatment tools. It is recommended that the reader observe this program at the Blount Hearing and Speech Center.

Cochlear Implant Program

The recent availability of cochlear implants has positively influenced the performance outcomes of both children and adults. It has especially demonstrated that young children, who are deaf, can benefit from an intensive auditory-based treatment. Because the Verbotonal Approach is auditory-based, it is a reasonable choice for a treatment program. The strategies and tools of the Verbotonal Approach are appropriate for developing listening skills and spoken language.

Early implantation, preceded by a pre-implant treatment program, is a high priority in developing a successful treatment program. Introducing vibrotactile speech input and the binaural headsets early on allows the young child to feel speech first. Then, the child will make a positive learning transfer from the Verbotonal Auditory Training Unit to his cochlear implant. After receiving the monaural implant, the vibratory speech input and a monaural headset on the child's contralateral ear is continued. This facilitates the development of binaural listening skills. The goal is to eventually have the child wear a monaural hearing aid on the contralateral ear. The binaural listening skills will help him in noisy environments (e.g., mainstreamed classroom). As the child develops better listening skills, the visual cues are reduced and the emphasis is placed on auditory-based input. These children are usually able to self-correct their speech errors through listening; they are considered "stars" by some educators. Most of these children do not need special education services and are mainstreamed at an early age.

Most children with a cochlear implant, however, do not make such rapid progress. They need an auditory-based program that develops both their listening skills and speech skills. For these children, natural visual cues (e.g., the clinician's face) are provided with the speech input; however, these visual cues are reduced as soon as possible to make the children focus on auditory speech input.

The Verbotonal strategy of error analysis and correction is important for all children. The children must be corrected regularly throughout the treatment program. The goal is to have each child develop self-correction skills, whereby he "hears" his speech error and makes the change to correct his speech production.

Most children with a cochlear implant are able to hear phonemes in the high-tonality zones (e.g., /i/ and /s/); however, some of the children will experience difficulty with the low-tonality phonemes (e.g., /u/ and /m/). This is why early Verbotonal treatment, before implantation, is so important. The pre-implant treatment helps the child develop his low-tonality auditory perception. Then, after the implant, both the low and high-tonality perception can develop simultaneously.

Cochlear implant mapping is usually based on the aided puretone audiogram and is not a functional evaluation of auditory speech recognition. This can produce significant problems for a child's auditory development. The Verbotonal clinician can avoid this problem by sharing the results of the Tonality Word Test with the audiologist. Then, the implant can be adjusted properly for both low and high-tonality perception.

Since a wide (broad) bandwidth is used with the Verbotonal Auditory Training Unit, it is ideal for the cochlear implant to also have a broad bandwidth. The Med El Implant uses a deep insertion of their electrode to stimulate a wide bandwidth. Following the Verbotonal wide-band speech stimulation, the Med El Implant may be most useful for the child. The continuation of wide-band speech stimulation should produce excellent speech recognition.

Because early detection of a hearing loss and early placement of a cochlear implant are so important, the parents and caregivers play a significant role in the child's development. The Verbotonal Approach is a parent-based program for both infants and toddlers. The parents can learn how to use vibratory speech input and binaural amplification. Parents are very capable of using body movements to correct the child's speech errors. The Verbotonal clinician provides intensive training for the parents in the early stages of treatment.

When parents are less available to work with their child, the Verbotonal clinician has to assume more responsibility for the child's auditory development. It may be necessary to provide treatment for this type of child in individual sessions or small groups. As the Verbotonal Approach to treatment is an auditory-based strategy, it can be applied to all children with cochlear implants. It can also be applied to adults with an implant. The consistent auditory input will maximize the child or adult's auditory speech perception.

Programs in Action: Verbotonal School and Clinic

International Verbotonal Programs

In 1954, Professor Petar Guberina adapted his foreign language strategy to serve children and adults with hearing impairments; it was named the Verbotonal Approach (also called System or Method). This Approach was used at the Hearing and Speech Center in Zagreb, Croatia. The center's staff includes speech, language, and hearing specialists, along with a medical team, to provide comprehensive services in both hearing and speech. These services include audiologic and medical diagnostics, preschool and school-age programs for deaf or hard-of-hearing children, treatment for adults with hearing impairments, hearing aid placement, vestibular testing, speech therapy with normal hearing children, and foreign language programs. In addition, the Verbotonal training unit with a headset, filters and vibrotactile speech output is used, so the clients could "hear" the target phoneme, and self-correct their speech error after hearing it.

In 1965, Professor Guberina was awarded a 5-year Verbotonal research grant from the U.S. Vocational Rehabilitation Department within Health, Education and Welfare (Guberina, 1972). This U.S. funding created an international interest in this Approach. The Zagreb Hearing and Speech Center and Zagreb University served as the education and training center for the international development of the Verbotonal Approach throughout the world; for example, Paskvalin

(1993) listed 1,300 published references in 11 different languages. Students and professionals attended workshops and completed practicum requirements to implement the Verbotonal approach in their country. The Approach included application with all communication problems, including teaching a foreign language.

Over the past 50 years (1954 to present), the International Verbotonal Association (IVTA) has provided research and clinical seminars, workshops, and symposiums on a regular basis. The IVTA also includes several national Verbotonal Associations, for example, Croatia, Italy, France, Spain, Russia, Japan, Brazil, Columbia, USA, and so forth. Most of these National Associations offer Verbotonal Training and Certification. For example, in the USA, the Verbotonal Association of the Americas offers Certification for an Implementer and for a Trainer, after passing a written and a practicum exam. The Certified Implementer has demonstrated competence in providing Verbotonal services, whereas the Certified Trainer is also competent in lecturing, supervising trainees, and may serve as a consultant.

Verbotonal Program in the United States

Following Verbotonal Training at The Ohio State University (1963–1967), Professor Asp applied for and was awarded a federally funded clinical research grant at The University of Tennessee in 1967. The overall goal was to evaluate the application of the Verbotonal Approach in the United States. The first task was to adapt the original Approach to an American University clinical model. The grant provided funds for extensive Verbotonal training through University courses, workshops, practicum, consultants from Zagreb, and the use of Verbotonal training units. The trained University staff of speech pathologists, audiologists, and teachers-of-the-deaf provided daily Verbotonal services for 40 preschool and school-age children who were deaf or hard-of-hearing. The staff also provided services for adults with hearing impairment, audiologic diagnostics, speech therapy for normal hearing clients, and courses for speaking a foreign language (e.g., Spanish, French, German, Japanese, Portuguese, and English as a second language). The Verbotonal Research Lab, established in 1967 at the University of Tennessee, has continued an ongoing clinical research program.

In 1975, the Hearing Service Program of the Knox County Public School adapted the Verbotonal University clinical model to a Verbotonal public school model (Asp et. al., 1990). This school model served children who were deaf or hard-of-hearing in the Knox County Public School System. The Verbotonal approach was incorporated into the regular school curriculum by using an Individualized Education Plan (IEP) for each child. The program goals were to maximize each child's listening and speaking skills, and to mainstream the children into regular classrooms. The children with lower skills started in a self-contained class at three years of age; the mainstreaming was increased gradually. The higher-level children began in full mainstreaming, with itinerant services. With the recent advances in cochlear implants, more children are beginning in full-time mainstreaming, if they have had an auditory-based birth-to-three-year treatment. The Knox County modification of Verbotonal Approach to a public-school model was accomplished, with the teachers and clinicians feeling comfortable with both the strategies and the tools. The parent plays an active role in the success of the program.

In 1984, Miami-Dade County Public Schools developed a Verbotonal program, using Knox County as a model (Strusinski, 1996). Certified Verbotonal Trainers from Knoxville have provided three one-week in-service workshops in Miami each year for their teachers and the clinicians. Both school systems have similar Verbotonal programs, and continue to interact to improve their quality of service. However, the difference is Miami-Dade is a large school system (500,000 total); whereas Knox is a small system (50,000 total). Their hearing-impaired caseload is 450 and 150, respectively. Both school systems continue providing Verbotonal services from preschool level through high school level.

Beginning in 1975, Verbotonal private-practice clinical models were developed. One of these models (Blount Hearing and Speech Center) offered birth-to-three-year services, elementary through high-school services and adult aural rehabilitation, services for normal hearing children with speech problems, and a hearing aid program that develops the client's perception through their residual hearing. This program has consistently received high hearing aid satisfaction from its clients. This clinical model continues to be used.

Free to Choose and Parent Involvement

Professionals or parents are free to choose some or all of the Verbotonal tools and strategies. The treatment tools can be adapted for use with other auditory-oral methods that are based on similar habilitation or rehabilitation strategies. The competence of the clinician, teacher, or parent is the most important factor in obtaining good listening skills with the children. This competence is enhanced by learning from the children, that is, what works and what does not work. Most successful clinicians and teachers continue to improve by sharing and discussing their results and insights with others. The clinical competence in an auditory-based strategy is difficult to master, therefore an ongoing effort is needed. In short, the Verbotonal Approach can be used in part or in full, and can be applied to a variety of communicative disorders or communication differences for both children and adults in school or clinical programs.

The invaluable role of the parent(s) or caretaker(s) in the development of all young children is well documented. The Verbotonal Approach always provides educational opportunities and encourages the parent(s) to be active in their child's development of listening, speaking, and language skills. This approach is adjusted to accommodate the availability and involvement of each parent. Certainly, the best results of the Verbotonal Approach come from the combined efforts and dedication of both the service provider(s) and the parent(s).

Summary

This book has presented the treatment strategy, tools, and the sequence of the Verbotonal Approach. It has stressed the link between the child's brain and the vestibular-auditory-speech modalities. The Verbotonal approach has been applied in both international and national clinical and school programs.

A well-trained teacher-clinician, competent in error analysis and speech modification, can implement this Approach utilizing the resources of a multidisciplinary team and a good individualized educational plan (IEP). It can be adapted to a classroom or individual sessions with infants, toddlers, or school-age children. For best results, the teachers and clinicians are encouraged to utilize all the treatment strategies and tools; however, they are free to choose those from which their children may benefit the most.

References

Asp, C. W., & Guberina, P. (1981). *Verbotonal method for rehabilitating people with communication problems.* New York: NY: World Rehabilitation Fund, Inc.

Asp, C. W., Kline, M., Duff, P. G., & Davis, C. (1990). Verbotonal method integrated into hearing services of Knox County School System, *SUVAG, 3,* 93–98.

Guberina, P. (1972). *The correlation between sensitivity of the vestibular system, and hearing and speech in Verbotonal rehabilitation* (Appendix 6, pp. 256–260).

Washington, DC: Office of Vocational Rehabilitation, Department of Health, Education, and Welfare.

Palmer, L. L. (1999). *Stimulating maturity through accelerated readiness training (SMART)*. Minneapolis, MN: Minnesota Learning Resource Center.

Paskvalin, M. (1993). *Bibliography of the Verbotonal system*. Zagreb, Croatia: Poliklinka SUVAG.

Rhodes, R. C. (1966). Discrimination of filtered CNC lists by normals and hypocusics. *The Journal of Auditory Research, 6*, 129–133.

Rook, L. (2005). Personal communication.

Strusinski, M. (1996). *Evaluation of the Verbotonal program*. [Report to the Office of Educational Accountability.] Miami, FL: Miami Dade Public Schools.

Glossary of Terms

accommodation: the ability of the eye to focus and quickly change focus from near to far and vice versa.

acoustic feature: distinctive feature that is based on the physical characteristics of the sound. For example, a sound that has a high-frequency hissing quality is characterized as sibilant.

acoustic property: perceptual characteristic of a sound that can be heard.

acuity: sharpness of slight measured with standard 20/20 vision charts.

adaptation: variation in the way in which articulators move and the extent to which vocal tract configuration changes shape according to preceding and following sounds.

adaptive response: an appropriate action in which the individual responds successfully to some environmental demand. Adaptive responses require good sensory integration, and they also further the sensory integrative process.

affricate: speech sound formed as a stop followed by a fricative release; a manner of articulation.

affrication: phonologic process in which fricatives are produced with a stop initiation.

allomorph: variation in the production of a meaningful segment that does not change its meaning, that is, plural markers can be produced as /s/, /z/, or /iz/.

allophone: articulatory gesture, or phone (speech sound), that is a variant of a phoneme category within the language. Allophones do not affect meaning.

alveolar: refers to speech sounds made with the tongue coming in contact with or moving close to the alveolar ridge; denotes place of articulation.

antecedent event: stimulus that immediately precedes the client's response.

anterior: refers to speech sounds in which the point of construction is anterior to the point for the production of /ʃ/; denotes place of articulation.

aphasia: acquired language disorder caused by brain damage, resulting in partial or complete impairment of language comprehension, formulation, and/or use in communication. The inability to speak and, sometimes, difficulty in understanding the spoken or written word.

apraxia: The lack of praxis or motor planning. When seen in children a sensory integrative dysfunction that interferes with planning and executing an unfamiliar task.

apraxia of speech: motor disorder of speech programming that may be characterized by inconsistent substitutions, oral searching behavior, greater articulatory breakdown in connected speech than in single sounds or words.

articulation: actions of the organs of speech that modify the breath stream resulting in speech sounds.

articulators: physical structures in the oral cavity that are responsible for or engaged in the production of speech sounds (i.e., lips, tongue, teeth, lower jaw, palate).

articulatory feature: distinctive feature that is based on the actions of the organs of speech. For example, front refers to a sound that is made in the front of the mouth.

aspirate: audible burst of air accompanying the opening of the closure after a stop.

assimilation: modification in the audible characteristics of a phone (speech sound) due to the characteristics of another phone in the utterance. An earlier phone in a word may affect a later phone, resulting in progressive assimilation, or a later phone may affect an earlier one, resulting in regressive assimilation. The phones do not need to be contiguous. Futhermore, the influencing phone may be deleted in the actual utterance.

assimilatory processes: phonologic processes that result from modification of one phoneme to match the characteristics of a neighboring phoneme.

auditory: Pertaining to the sense of hearing; related to or experienced through hearing.

augmentative communication: any approach designed to support, enhance, or augment the communication of individuals who cannot use speech for independent verbal communication in all situations.

autism: a form of brain disorder affecting the child's ability to relate to people, things, and events.

awareness of sound: the detection of sound (speech) through the perception of on-off, long-short, or loud-soft distinctions.

babbling: prespeech behavior characterized by syllables that may be initiated or terminated by consonantlike sounds.

back: refers to speech sounds made with the tongue retracted; denotes place of articulation.

backing: phonologic process in which posterior consonants are substituted for anterior ones.

baseline: record of the rate of a behavior before training or conditioning procedures are initiated.

behavioral probe: sample of the client's behavior as measured by a testing procedure.

bifid uvula: division or cleft in the small oval-shaped process extending from the lower border of the velum at midline.

bilabial: refers to speech sounds made with partial or complete closure of the lips or of the lips and teeth; denotes place of articulation.

binocular: of, relating to, using, or adapted to the use of both eyes.

binocularity: the simultaneous use of the two eyes in the act of vision.

body as a resonator: the whole body is involved in the perception of speech. The larger body parts (i.e., the abdomen) respond to the lower frequencies in the speech signal, and the smaller body parts (i.e., head) respond to the higher frequencies. Perception by the whole body becomes accentuated when the most efficient perception (the auditory system) is impaired.

body as a transmitter: the whole body is involved in producing (transmitting) speech, which includes both the tensions and the movements of the body and the speech articulators. It is presumed that the state of the body affects the state of the articulators.

body movements: see *movement therapy.*

body percept: a person's perception of his own body. It consists of sensory pictures or "maps" of the body stored in the brain. May also be called body scheme, body image, or neuronal of the body.

brachiation: to progress by swinging from one hold to another by arms.

brainstem: the lowest and innermost portion of the brain. The brainstem contains nuclei that regulate internal organic functions, arousal of the nervous system as a whole, and elementary sensory-motor processing.

brain transfer: the ability of a hearing-impaired person to identify phonemes through a restricted frequency response (OFR) even though some of the phonemes are outside this frequency band. This ability is learned through training and natural experience. Transfer is a central process of the brain. Transfer can be tested with Verbotonal audiometry, and used to explain the errors on a perceptual continuum.

carryover: in articulation training, the ability to use a target sound during functional speech outside the therapy setting.

categorical perception: listener's classification of a speech sound as belonging to a specific phonologic category. A unit of speech is not classified as belonging partially to one category and partially to another, but categorically to a single category.

central programming: the neural functions that are innate within our central nervous system; they do not have to be learned. Creeping on hands and knees and walking are good examples of centrally programmed actions.

cerebellum: the part of the brain that is wrapped around the back of the brainstem. It processes proprioceptive and vestibular sensations to help make body movements accurate. It also processes all other types of sensation.

cerebral cortex: the outer layer of the cerebral hemispheres. It includes areas for very precise sensory processing, especially of visual and auditory details and sensations from the body. It also executes fine, voluntary body movements and speech. It is concerned with thoughts, mental evaluations, and goals.

cerebral hemispheres: the two large sections of the brain that lie over and around the brainstem. The hemispheres continue the sensory processing that begins at lower levels and assist in producing voluntary motor responses and behavior.

cerebral palsy: developmental disability in which the main clinical feature is lack of motor control.

cleft palate: structural anomaly that can affect the tissues, muscles, and bony processes of lip, alveolar process, hard palate, and uvula.

cluster reduction: phonologic process in which one or more members of a consonant cluster are omitted (i.e., /pr/ for /spr/ or /b/ for /bl/).

coalescence: form of assimilation that occurs when the features of two sounds are combined to form a third sound; also called reciprocal assimilation.

coarticulation: the simultaneous movement of the muscles and articulators to produce two different phones in connected speech. This movement modifies the production of adjacent phones.

cocontraction: the simultaneous contraction of all the muscles around a joint to stabilize it.

cognates: two sounds made with the same place and manner of articulation, differing only in whether they are voiced or unvoiced (e.g., /t,d/, /f,v/).

communication: process of encoding, transmitting, and decoding signals in order to exchange information and ideas between participants.

compensatory speech production: substitution of a perceptually similar phoneme for a phoneme that cannot be produced normally by the speaker.

consequent event: stimulus that immediately follows the client's response.

consonant: speech sound made by marked or complete constriction in the vocal tract. Consonants may initiate and terminate syllables.

consonant cluster: two or more adjacent consonants occurring within the same syllable.

consonant harmony: phonologic process in which the production of one consonant is modified to match the characteristics of another consonant in the utterance

consonant sequence: two or more consonants not separated by a vowel; the two consonants can cross syllable boundaries. See *consonant cluster* for comparison.

consonant singleton: single consonant separated from other consonants by a vowel or silence

continuant: refers to speech sounds that can be maintained in a steady state; denotes distinctive feature.

contrastive items: speech sound pairs of which one sound is the target sound and the other is the error sound.

convergence: the act of turning the two eyes inward and focusing on an object as it moves toward a person.

conversational juncture: in articulation training, the transitional between words in conversational speech.

coronal: refers to speech sounds made with the tongue blade raised; denotes distinctive feature.

cranial nerves: the set of nerves running from the head and face directly to the brain (without passing through the spinal cord) and from the brain back to the head and face.

cue: hints or suggestions provided to the client to assist in the production of the correct response..

cycle: time periods during which all deficient phonologic patterns are targeted in succession.

deaffriction: phonologic process in which affricates are produced without the stop initiation or without the fricative release.

deep test: an articulation test designed to identify phonetic contexts in which a target speech sound is produced incorrectly as well as those in which it is produced correctly (facilitating contexts). The target sound is assessed in a variety of phonetic environments.

dental prosthesis: artificial device that substitutes for missing teeth and maintains correct dentition.

dentition: form and arrangement of the teeth in the dental arch.

devoicing: phonologic process in which voiceless sounds are substituted for voiced sounds.

diadochokinetic rate: rate of movement of the articulators (tongue, lips, etc.) as measured by ability to repeat syllables rapidly.

diffuse: refers to speech sounds produced forward in the oral cavity including labials, dental, and alveolars in contrast to palatals and velars; denotes distinctive feature.

diphthong: vowel created by a change in the configuration of the vocal tract during vowel production that alters the resonating characteristic of the tract. Two vowels are fused together within a single syllable.

directionality: understanding the concepts of up-down, left-right, back-front, and so forth as projected in space. Laterality, or the knowledge of left and right on oneself is the basis for directionality.

dissimilation: phonologic process in which one of two similar sounds is produced in a manner to make it less similar.

distinctive feature: articulatory or acoustic element that defines a phoneme. Each phoneme can be thought of as a unique combination of features.

distributed: refers to the length of the construction of the vocal tract that exceeds the narrow construction produced by the teeth for /f/, /v/, /θ/, and /ð/; denotes distinctive feature.

duration: the time during which something exists or lasts.

dysarthria: faulty production of speech caused by nervous system damage. It may involve impairment of resonation, articulation, phonation, or prosody.

dyspraxia: poor praxis or motor planning. A less severe, but more common dysfunction than apraxia.

ear training: see *sensory perceptual training.*

epenthesis: insertion of a sound between two others. This insertion would generally make the sequence easier to say (e.g., /warmpθ/ for warmth.

error analysis and correction: analyzing the responses (speech) of the child according to perceptual speech parameters and then modifying the next stimulus to improve and/or correct the next response.

    a. Indirect correction might involve movement therapy to establish the correct movement of the speech articulators. At this phase, the child is unaware of the correct. This helps him maintain the natural flow of speech and does not develop inhibition for speaking.

    b. Direct correction is used after the child has developed vocal control and the natural flow of speech. The child is aware of the correction. Most of this type of correction is done in individual therapy.

expression of emotions: a training technique using the emotions of the child to evoke spontaneous speech and perception.

extension: the action of straightening the neck, back, arms, or legs.

extinction: return of a response that has been conditioned using positive reinforcement to its preconditioned rate (base rate) after the reinforcer has been eliminated.

eye-hand coordination: the ability of the eye and hand to work together to complete a task.

facilitating context: phonetic environment in which a sound usually produced incorrectly is more easily produced correctly.

facilitation: a neural process that promotes the conduction of impulses or a response to them. Facilitation is the opposite of inhibition.

far point acuity: sharpness of vision at 20 feet or blackboard distance.

feedback: in articulation training, the sensory (auditory, visual, tactile, or kinesthetic) information that is utilized to monitor the production of speech.

fixation: aiming or directing the eyes while shifting rapidly from one object to another, such as reading from word to word on a line or copying from a textbook to a notebook.

fixed ratio schedule of reinforcement: reinforcers provided following a fixed number of responses, that is, one reinforcer following every correct response, or every third correct response, or whatever number is chosen.

flexion: the act of bending or pulling in a part of the body.

flowchart: taxonomy of objectives arranged from easy to more difficult.

frequency: the number of repetitions of a process in a unit of time..

fricative: consonant produced by forcing the voiced or voiceless breath stream through a constriction formed in the vocal tract. Turbulence in the airstream produces friction noise or aperiodic sound.

fronting: phonologic process in which sounds are produced farther forward in the oral cavity (usually at the alveolar ridge) than for the standard production.

fusion: abinocular response that simultaneously combines the separate inputs from the two eyes into a single mental image at the brain level.

glide: prevocalic consonant characterized by a rapid movement of the articulators from a high front or back tongue arch to a vowel that follows. Although glides are resonants, they are also considered to be consonants because they initiate syllables.

gliding: phonologic process in which glides are substituted for another class of sounds (usually liquids).

global: presenting speech in a natural way so that all the acoustic parameters are present.

glottal: refers to speech sounds made by closure of the vocal folds with no characteristic resononant shape of the vocal tract; denotes place of articulation.

glottal replacement: phonologic process in which consonants are replaced by the glottal stop.

grave: refers to speech sounds made at the very front (/p/, /b/, /m/) or the very back (/k/, /g/, /ŋ/) of the oral cavity; denotes distinctive feature.

gravitational insecurity: an abnormal anxiety and distress caused by inadequate modulation or inhibition of sensations that arise when the gravity receptors of the vestibular system are stimulated by head position or movement.

haptic: tactile-kinesthetic sensation.

high: refers to sounds made with the body of the tongue elevated above the neutral position; denotes distinctive feature.

holistic: emphasizing the organic of functional relation between parts and wholes.

homonym: word that sounds the same as another word, but has a different meaning.

homorganic: two phones produced at the same place of articulation.

hyperactivity: excessively or pathologically active.

hypernasal tone: excessive nasal resonance during phonation.

inhibition: a neural process that reduces the conductivity of certain synapses so that some impulses are blocked. Inhibition performs an important function by reducing excess neural activity. Unlike in other fields of psychology, the neurologic term "inhibition" does not have a negative connotation.

instructional objective: written statement describing the desired behavior, the conditions under which the behavior should occur, and the degree of accuracy of the behavior; synonymous with behavioral objective.

intelligibility: degree to which speech is understood by others.

intensity: the magnitude of force or energy per unit saturation.

interauditory discrimination: client's comparison of his own auditory image of the target sound with someone else's production (usually the clinician's during the discrimination phase of sensory perceptual training).

interrupted: refers to speech sounds in which the airstream is completely blocked at some point during production; denotes distinctive feature.

intervocalic: between two vowels.

intra-auditory discrimination: client's comparison of his auditory image of the target sound with his or her own production during the discrimination phase of sensory perceptual training.

intraoral breath pressure: buildup of air within the oral cavity. This air pressure creates the force necessary for the expulsion of air for plosive sounds.

jargon: prespeech behavior characterized by connected syllables produced with adult-like intonation patterns.

kinesthetic: sense of position or movement of articulatory structures.

labiodental: refers to speech sounds made with the lower lip and upper teeth; denotes place of articulation.

labyrinth: from the Greek work for "maze." The complex bony structure of the inner ear. It contains both the vestibular and auditory receptors.

lateral: refers to speech sounds in which the midline is constricted so that the air escapes around the sides of the tongue; denotes distinctive feature.

lateral coordination: the horizontal balance of the eyes.

laterality: the internal awareness of the two sides of the body and their labels of left and right. This serves as a motoric basis for making directional (left, right) judgments in space (e.g., letter reversals).

lateralization: the tendency for certain processes to be handled more efficiently on one side of the brain than the other. In most people, the right hemisphere becomes more efficient in processing spatial and musical patterns, while the left hemisphere specializes in verbal and logical processes.

lax: refers to speech sounds made with relatively less muscle tension and shorter duration; denotes distinctive feature.

learning: a change in neural function as a consequence of experience.

learning disorder: a difficulty in learning to read, write, compute, or do schoolwork that cannot be attributed to impaired sight or hearing, to mental retardation or to poor motivation.

limbic system: the parts of the cerebral hemispheres concerned with emotionally based behavior and emotional response to sensory input. The limbic system receives and processes input from all sensory channels.

linguadental: refers to speech sounds made with the tongue touching or moving close to the teeth; denotes place of articulation.

lingual: refers to speech sounds made with the tongue as one of the articulators; denotes place of articulation.

linguistics: the study of language.

liquid: consonant for which the articulators make only partial, frictionless approximation (/r/ and /l/); also called *semivowel.*

liquid simplification: phonologic process in which liquids are produced as glides; also called *gliding of liquids.*

locomotion: movement of the body from one place to another.

logarithmic graph: graph that uses equal intervals to record rate of response.

low: refers to sounds made with the tongue lowered; denotes distinctive feature.

maintenance: in articulation training, retention of correct production of a target sound or pattern after the course of therapy is complete.

malocclusion: abnormal relationship between the upper and lower teeth.

manner of articulation: the way the breath stream is modified to produce a speech sound (e.g., fricative or stop).

marked: the value of a feature (usually the plus value) that presumably makes a sound more difficult to produce.

meaningful context: in articulation training, a speech production that resembles one used in real communication

melodic intonation therapy: therapy approach for aphasia that uses exaggerated intonation patterns to help the patient produce fluent speech.

metalinguistics: the branch of linguistics that deals with ability to think and talk about language.

metathesis: transposition of two adjacent sounds (e.g., /æks/ for ask).

migration: phonologic process in which a sound is moved to another position in the word.

minimal pair: two different words (i.e., different meanings) that differ by only one phoneme or one distinctive feature.

modulation: the brain's regulation of its own activity. Modulation involves facilitating some neural messages to produce more of a perception or response, and inhibiting other messages to reduce excess or extraneous activity.

monocular: involving or affecting a single eye.

morpheme: smallest unit of language that has meaning.

morphophonemics: study of the rules that govern the production of sounds in combination of morphemes. These rules relate phonologic rules and syntactic rules.

motor: pertaining to body movement or posture.

motor control system: central nervous system motor encoding system involved in the planning of articulation.

motor execution system: parts of the nervous, muscular, and skeletal systems involved in the production of speech sounds.

motor planning: the ability of the brain to conceive of, organize, and carry out a sequence of unfamiliar actions. Also known as praxis.

movement therapy: movements of the body for the purpose of stimulating and/or correcting the movements of the speech articulators. Other terms that are used interchangeably are body movements, macro movements, and large body movements.

multisensory: refers to presenting the stimulus (speech) under conditions that allow all possible clues from auditory, visual, tactile, propioceptive, and kinesthetic channels. Ability to stimulate using taste, smell, visual, auditory, and tactile pathways.

multisyllabic words: words with more than one syllable.

muscular generalization: the state or condition in which a muscle or muscle group affects adjacent muscles. For example, an increase in body muscle tension that generalizes and increases the muscle tension of the speech articulators.

nasal: consonant in which the air resonates in the nasopharynx while the oral cavity is blocked. The velopharyngeal port is open making nasal resonance possible for the sounds /m, n, ŋ/.

nasal resonance: modification of the glottal tone resulting from the coupling of the nasal tract with the vocal tract when the velum is lowered.

near point acuity: sharpness of vision at 16 inches or reading distance.

neurogenic: originating within the nervous system.

neuron: the structural and functional unit of the nervous system. It consists of a cell body with terminals for receiving nerve impulses and a fiber capable of sending impulses.

nuclei: a cluster of nerve cell bodies that organize and integrate sensory and motor activity. In a way, they are "business centers" for the operations of the brain.

nystagmus: a series of automatic, back-and-forth eye movements. Different conditions produce this reflex. A common way of producing it is by an abrupt stop following a series of rotations of the body. The duration and regularity of postrotary nystagmus are some of the indicators of vestibular system efficiency.

obstruent: consonant produced by creating airstream turbulence within the oral cavity. Obstruents include voiced and voiceless stops, fricatives, and affricates.

occlusion: relationship between the upper and lower teeth.

occupational therapy: a profession that employs a purposeful activity to help the client form adaptive responses that enable the nervous system to work more efficiently.

open syllable: syllable that ends in a vowel, not terminated by a consonant, for example, "to, saw, lie, " and so forth.

optimal frequency response (OFR): the frequency responses that produce the best response (speech) for the child or adult for this particular stage of learning (progression). The auditory training unit and/or hearing aid is set for the OFR for training and usually corresponds to the most sensitive area of hearing for the client. With the proper training, hearing-impaired people can learn to identify phonemes thought to be outside the frequency range of their hearing.

optimal octave: the octave bandwidth that produces the highest identification score for a particular speech sound (phoneme). This filtered phoneme sounds similar to the same phoneme when it is not filtered. For example, /i/ filtered through 3200 to 6400 sounds like the unfiltered /i/. The optimal octaves are based on the perception of a group of normal hearing listeners.

optimum: see *optimum learning condition.*

optimum learning condition: the stimulus and/or condition that produces the best possible responses (speech) from the child or adult for their particular stage of learning (progression).

oral apraxia: inability to perform oral vegetative movements such as blowing, chewing, protruding the tongue, or licking the lips voluntarily upon request.

organic articulation disorders: disorders that arise from physical anomalies affecting structure or function of the mechanisms of speech.

oronasal fistula: small opening in the hard palate.

palatal: refers to speech sounds that are made with the body of the tongue touching or moving close to the hard palate; denotes place of articulation.

palatogram: impressions made by the tongue during speech sound production on an artificial palate that is covered with chalk or powder and inserted into the mouth.

paraphasia: articulatory error resulting from difficulty with phonological and grammatical rules; also called paraphasic error.

paresis: partial paralysis or muscular weakness.

percept or perception: the meaning the brain gives to sensory input. Sensations are objective; perception is subjective.

perceptual continuum: the arrangement of the 43 phonemes of American English as a continuum from the low to the high pitch (tonality) for the purpose of analyzing segmental (phonemic) errors and using the continuum as a reference and strategy for correction.

perceptual speech parameters: the method of analyzing the suprasegmental and segmental parts of the speech signal by reference to the perceptual references (parameters) of pitch, loudness, duration, tension, pause, intonation, and rhythm.

pharyngeal fricative: friction sound created by constriction of the airstream between the tongue and pharyngeal wall or by constriction of the pharynx.

pharyngeal plosive: sound created by the explosive release of a complete construction between the tongue and pharyngeal wall.

phonation: the production of voice by the vibration of the vocal folds.

phone: speech sound segment identified as a member of a particular phoneme or representing a specific phoneme.

phoneme: group of phones that are perceived as belonging to the same sound category. The set of phonemes are considered to constitute the discrete speech units of a language. Also, a speech sound (segment) that is unique to a particular language.

phonemic rhythms: the combination of movement therapy and speech rhymes.

phonetic environment: the other speech sounds surrounding a given phoneme within a word or syllable.

phonetic feature: attributes of a sound that can be expressed in acoustic or physiologic terms.

phonetics: the branch of phonology that deals with individual speech sounds, their production, and their representation by written symbols.

phonological knowledge: information that is an underlying representation of a phonologic/articulation unit.

phonologic pattern: standard adult speech pattern of a linguistic community.

phonologic process: patterned modification of speech sound production away from the standard adult production. Phonologic processes usually simplify the syllable structure /s/ or phoneme classes.

phonology: the study of linguistic rules governing the sound system of the language, including speech sounds, speech sound production, and the combination of sounds in meaningful utterances.

phonotactics: rules for allowable sound combinations in syllables.

place of articulation: the location of the vocal tract constriction for production of a speech sound.

positive reinforcer: stimulus that immediately follows a response and increases the rate of the response.

posterior: primary place of articulation in back of oral cavity or in glottal area.

postural background movements: the subtle, spontaneous body adjustments that make overt movements of the hands, such as reaching for a distant object, easier. These postural adjustments depend upon good integration of vestibular and proprioceptive inputs.

postvocalic: following the vowel in a syllable.

pragmatics: the use of language in society.

praxis: see *motor planning.*

preparatory set: voluntary and/or reflexive preparation of an organism to respond in a particular way to anticipated stimuli. In speech, preparatory set may include the combined respiratory, phonatory, and articulatory systems. In articulation, anticipation of upcoming sounds results in alteration of articulatory postures and movements.

prevocalic: preceding the vowel in a syllable.

production training: phase of articulation training designed to elicit and establish a new sound pattern that will replace the client's error pattern.

programmed instruction: instructional procedure in which the author has written a systematic set of instructions to be presented to the client. Feedback regarding accuracy of the responses to these instruction is provided.

progression: the stages of learning a child must experience to develop good speech, language, and listening skills. Each stage is affected by and dependent on the previous stages. The optimum (ideal) conditions for learning change at each level of this progression.

prompt: exact model of the correct response.

prone: the body position with the face and stomach downward.

proprioception: from the Latin word for "one's own." The sensations from the muscles and joints. Proprioceptive input tells the brain when and how the muscles are contracting or stretching, and when and how the joints are bending, extending, or being pulled or compressed. This information enables the brain to know where each part of the body is and how it is moving.

protective extension: the reflex that extends the arms to provide protection when the body is falling.

punisher: stimulus that immediately follows a response and results in a decrease in the rate of the response.

readiness skills: fundamental skills needed to succeed in school.

receptor: a cell or group of cells that are sensitive to some type of sensory energy. Receptors transform the sensation into electrical impulses and send them over sensory nerves to the spinal cord or brain.

reduplicated babbling: prespeech behavior characterized by combinations of identical or similar syllables.

reduplication: phonologic process in which different syllables are produced similarly.

reflex: an innate and automatic response to sensory input. We have reflexes to withdraw from pain, startle at sensations that surprise us, and extend our head and body upward in response to vestibular input. There are many other reflexes.

response cost: immediate removal of a previously acquired reinforcer following an incorrect response.

reticular core: the central core of the brainstem, and one of the most complex and entangled portions of the brain. Every sensory system sends impulses to the reticular core, which then sends influences to the rest of the brain.

retroflex: refers to sound made with the tip of the tongue curled back; denotes distinctive feature.

round: refers to speech sounds made with the lips rounded; denotes distinctive feature.

rule: statement that describes some aspect of the language. Phonologic rules describe the sound system of the language.

saccadic: a small, rapid, jerky movement of the eye as it jumps from fixation on one point to another (as in reading).

schedule of reinforcement: a schedule the clinician experimenter devises to determine how frequently a reinforcer will be provided following the correct response.

schemata: structured memories of related perceptual, conceptual, social, emotional, and physical information derived from interactions with the environment. Existing schemata are used to process and organize new information.

script: schemata for a series of actions or event. These generalized episodes or routine activities form the basis for semantic knowledge and the ability to participate appropriately in old and new situations.

secondary reinforcer: stimulus that has been paired with a primary reinforcer (conditioned) and acquires the same or similar effect upon rate of response as the primary reinforcer.

segmentals: the individual speech sounds or phonemes of a language which include vowels, diphthongs, and consonants. Perceptually, each segment (phoneme) is identified by a phonetic symbol and is restricted by that brief time interval. Segmentals are different from the suprasegmentals.

self-esteem: the way one sees oneself.

semantics: meaning in language.

semivowel: speech sound made by a movement from one vocal tract shape to another in a manner similar to diphthongs. Although semivowels are resonants, they are considered to be consonants because they initiate syllables. Also called *liquids* or *glides*.

sensory input: the streams of electrical impulses flowing from the sense receptors in the body to the spinal cord and brain.

sensory integration: the organization of sensory input for use. The "use" may be a perception of the body or the world, or an adaptive response, or a learning process, or the development of some neural function. Through sensory integration, the many parts of the nervous system work together so that a person can interact with the environment effectively and experience appropriate satisfaction.

sensory integrative dysfunction: an irregularity or disorder in brain function that makes it difficult to integrate sensory input. Sensory integrative dysfunctions are the basis for many, but not all, learning disorders.

sensory integrative therapy: treatment involving sensory stimulation and adaptive responses to it according to the child's neurologic needs. Therapy usually involves full body movements that provide vestibular proprioceptive, and tactile stimulation. It usually does not involve activities at a desk, speech training, reading lessons, or training in specific perceptual or motor skills. The goal of therapy is to improve the way the brain processes and organizes sensations.

sensory perceptual training: technique used in articulation training that emphasizes the development of an auditory model to serve as an internal standard against which comparison of speech sound production can be made.

shaping: establishing a target behavior (speech sound) by reinforcing successively closer approximations to the target until correct production is achieved.

sibilant: fricative with a high frequency hissing quality (/s,z,ʃ,ʒ/).

sight: the ability to see and the eyes response to light shining into it.

situational play or teaching: creating a real or imaginary situation that is meaningful and provokes spontaneous speech from the children. This technique is used to establish meaning which results in improved language skills.

sonorant: refers to speech sounds that allow the airstream to pass unimpeded through the oral or nasal cavity; denotes distinctive feature. Phonemes include vowels, nasals, glides, and liquids.

Southern California Sensory Integration Tests (SCSIT): a series of tests designed to assess the status of sensory integration or its dysfunction.

specialization: in general, the process by which one part of the brain becomes more efficient at particular functions. Most specialized functions are lateralized, that is, one side of the brain is more proficient in the function than the other side.

speech: dynamic neuromuscular process of producing sounds for transmitting verbal messages.

speech rhymes: short speech rhymes for the purpose of developing propioceptive and auditory memory span for rhymes are usually four lines in 2/2 or 4/4 time and range from simple syllable sequences to complex forms containing meaningful words. Other terms that are used interchangeably are speech rhythms, musical rhythms, rhythmic stimulation, and rhymes.

speech sound discrimination: identification of a sound or a comparison between two sounds. Usually the listener is asked to name a sound or indicate whether two sounds are the same or different.

stabilization: phase of articulation training designed to develop the client's ability to produce the target sound easily and quickly.

stereoscope: a piece of equipment used for binocular vision training.

stimulability: ability of a client to correctly produce a target phoneme by imitating the clinician's exaggerated model.

stimulation: in the earlier stages of training, the child is stimulated with speech and body movements to increase his ability to vocalize and to strengthen the link between the stimulus and responses. At this stage, the clinician does not correct the child's responses.

stimulus generalization: occurrence of a response, once it is conditioned to a specific stimulus, in the presence of stimuli that are similar.

stimulus-response model: a training model in which the clinician presents a stimulus (speech) and the child or adult responds by imitating the stimulus. The clinician analyzes the response and either presents the same stimulus or modifies the next stimulus for improving and/or correcting the response.

stop: manner of articulation characterized by complete stoppage of the airstream.

stopping: phonologic process in which stops are substituted for continuants.

stridency deletion: phonologic process in which the stridency associated with fricative or affricate sounds is deleted. The resulting sound will usually be a stop or glide. Stridency deletion cannot occur alone without some other modification of the sound.

strident: refers to speech sounds in which noise is produced by forceful airflow striking the back of the teeth (sibilants and /f/ and /v/); denotes distinctive feature.

structure: unique arrangement of the seven parameters for the clinician's stimulus or a response that can be analyzed by the clinician by determining the amount or magnitude of each parameter.

submucous cleft: cleft of the soft or hard palate in which the surface mucosal tissues are connected, while the underlying bone or muscle tissues are separated.

substitution processes: phonologic processes that modify the characteristics of a phoneme resulting in the substitution of one phoneme for another.

suprasegmentals: changes in the spoken speech signal that are not restricted to one phoneme or speech sound (i.e., an upward inflection that extends over all the syllables of the utterance). The suprasegmentals provide the structure for all phonemes and can be described as rhythm and intonation.

syllable: speech unit consisting of one vowel. The consonants that may surround this vowel are determined by phonotactic rules.

syllable reduction: phonologic process in which a syllable in a multisyllabic word is deleted.

syllable structure process: phonologic process that modifies the shape of a syllable. Examples include omission or addition of a phoneme or eliminating the syllable altogether.

synapse: the place where two neurons make electrochemical contact and also the transmission of a nerve impulse from one neuron to the next. Neural impulses travel a path of many synapses, and each synapse adds to the processing of those impulses.

syntax: rules of language that govern the arrangement and sequence of words according to the meaning relationships among them.

systematic phonetic level: abstract phonetic information that provides direction for the motor control system in articulation.

tactile: related to or experience through sense of touch or feeling.

tactile defensiveness: a sensory integrative dysfunction in which tactile sensations cause excessive emotional reactions, hyperactivity, or other behavior problems.

target behavior: desired response the clinician wishes to obtain.

target phoneme: error phoneme that is the principal focus of treatment. The phoneme that is the principal focus of treatment. The phoneme may represent a target pattern and thus be used to facilitate the development of the pattern.

target pattern: adult sound class, syllable shape, or syllable sequence that is the focus of treatment.

telebinocular: an instrument used to test vision.

tense: refers to sounds made with a relatively greater degree of muscle tension and longer duration; denotes distinctive feature.

time out: removal of a subject from conditions in which the subject could receive positive reinforcement.

tonality: the pitch of individual speech sounds (phonemes) whereby /i/ is perceived as higher in pitch than /a/, and /s/ is higher than /b/. The pitch or tonality can be described as the spectral pitch, and associated with the timbre of phonemes.

tonic neck reflex: the reflex that makes an arm tend to extend when the head is turned toward that arm. The other arm tends to flex at the same time. It should be integrated into the overall function of the brain by the first few months of life, but remains overly active in many children with brain dysfunctions.

tracking: the ability of the eyes to move smoothly from one point to another. Example: following words on a page from left to right.

tract: a long, thin bundle of nerve fibers that carry sensory input or motor responses from one place in the nervous system to another.

transfer: extension of learned behavior from the original setting (i.e., treatment) to other settings.

unaided condition: presenting speech to the client without any amplification. The training unit, hearing aid, or cochlear implant is not used. Unaided is a reference condition.

unaspirated: stop made without an audible burst of air accompanying the opening of the closure.

underlying phonologic form: an abstract representation from which the actual production can be derived by application of phonologic rules.

variable ratio schedule of reinforcement: reinforcers provided following an average (not fixed) number of correct responses. For example, on a variable ratio schedule of 3, the client might receive a reinforcer after 2 correct responses, another reinforcer after 4 correct responses, and so forth. The average number of reinforcers is one per 3 correct responses.

variegated babbling: prespeech behavior characterized by connected syllables produced with adult-like intonation patterns; also called jargon.

velar: refers to sounds made by the tongue touching or moving close to the soft palate (velum); denotes place articulation.

velopharyngeal closure: movement of the velum and pharynx to close off or separate the nasal cavity from the oral cavity, thus directing airflow through the mouth rather than through the nose.

velopharyngeal incompetence: inability to achieve adequate separation of the nasal cavity from the oral cavity by action of the velum and the pharynx when the structures appear normal. Excessive nasal resonance may result.

Verbotonal Training Unit: the vibrotactile and acoustic filters unit that is used for training the child or adult in the classroom and/or individual therapy.

vertical coordination: the up-and-down balance of the eyes.

vestibular: pertaining to the functions of the inner ear dealing with posture, equilibrium, muscular tones and orientation in environmental space.

Vestibular-Auditory Training Unit: see *Verbotonal Training Unit.*

vestibular-bilateral disorder: a sensory integrative dysfunction caused by underreactive vestibular responses. It is characterized by shortened durations of nystagmus, poor integration of the two sides of the body and brain, and difficulty in learning to read or compute.

vestibular nerve: the fibers of the eighth cranial nerve that carry vestibular input from the gravity receptors and semicircular canals to the vestibular nuclei.

vestibular nuclei: the groups of cells in the brainstem that process vestibular sensory input and send it on to other brain locations for organization of a response. These complex "business centers" also integrate vestibular input with input from other sensory channels.

vestibular receptors: the sense organs that detect the pull of gravity and the movements of the head. They are located in the labyrinth of the inner ear. Each inner ear contains gravity receptors in tiny sacs and movement receptors in semicircular canals.

vestibular-spinal tract: The pathways for neural messages from vestibular nuclei to the motor neutrons in the spinal cord. Vestibular-spinal messages help to maintain muscle tone, hold the body upright, and keep the joints extended.

vestibular system: the sensory system that responds to the position of the head in relation to gravity and accelerated or decelerated movement.

vibrator: it is placed on the client's body (hand, wrist, leg, or head), so the client can feel the clinician's and his or her vocal patterns of speech. The surface of the vibrator moves with the same precision as a diaphram in an earphone. The vibrator is used with a *Verbotonal Training Unit.*

Vibro-sounding board: a smooth board that is large enough for the child to lay or sit on; he feels the vibrations of his and the clinician's speech. As the clinician speaks into the microphone, the vibrators activate the entire vibrating board..

vibrotactile input: the tactile sensation that a client perceives through a vibrator that is attached to or held in his hand or fingers, body or head, or is attached to a Vibro-Board.

vision: the result of the child's ability to interpret and understand the information that comes to the child through her or his eyes.

visual: pertaining to the sense of sight.

vocable: prespeech utterance produced with a phonetically consistent form in a given context. A vocable is not a true word because it is not based on an adult word.

vocalic: referring to vowels.

vocalization: 1. phonologic process in which consonants (usually glides or liquids) are produced as vowels; also called vowelization. 2. nonverbal utterance.

voice onset time: the difference in time between the release of a stop and the onset of voicing.

voiced: refers to speech sounds in which the vocal folds vibrate; denotes distinctive feature.

voiceless: sounds in which the vocal folds do not vibrate.

voicing: phonologic process in which voicing is added to voiceless sounds.

vowel: speech sound made with an open vocal tract. Vowels constitute syllables and are therefore also termed syllabics.

Index